HEADACHE HELP

HEADACHE HELP

A COMPLETE GUIDE TO
UNDERSTANDING HEADACHES
AND THE MEDICINES THAT
RELIEVE THEM

FULLY REVISED AND UPDATED

LAWRENCE ROBBINS, M.D., AND SUSAN S. LANG

Houghton Mifflin Company

BOSTON   NEW YORK

2000

Visit our Web site: www.hmco.com/trade.

Library of Congress Cataloging-in-Publication Data

Robbins, Lawrence D.
Headache help : a complete guide to understanding headaches
and the medicines that relieve them / Lawrence Robbins and
Susan S. Lang.—Rev. and updated.
         p.   cm.
ISBN 0-618-04436-1
1. Headache—Popular works.   I. Lang, Susan S.   II. Title.
RB128.R628   2000   616.8'491—dc21   00-036940

Book design by Anne Chalmers

Printed in the United States of America

QUM 10 9 8 7 6 5 4 3 2 1

The information presented in case histories and stories in *Headache Help* is medically
accurate. However, all names, places, and identifying characteristics have been changed to
protect privacy. Some case histories contain elements from more than one patient. Any re-
semblance to persons living or dead is coincidental.

For my family
and those suffering
the burden of head pain

— L.D.R.

For Solon J. Lang

— S.S.L.

THE GRIEF OF THE HEAD
IS THE GRIEF OF GRIEFS.
— James Howell,
English Proverbs, 1659

Visit our Web site, www.headachedrugs.com, to keep abreast of the latest headache information. Here you'll find a vast amount of headache-related material, starting with our links:

What's New?
Patient's Corner
Medications
General Advice
Headache Books
Headache Herbs

CONTENTS

· · · · · · · · · ·

Preface   xiii

1. Understanding the Modern Approach   1
2. Helping Yourself   18
3. Being a Good Health Consumer   42
4. Recognizing Migraines   55
5. Treating Migraines in Progress   64
6. Preventing Migraines   94
7. Women, Hormones, and Migraines   129
8. Treating Tension Headaches in Progress   142
9. Preventing Tension Headaches   152
10. Understanding and Treating Cluster Headaches   171
11. Headaches in Children and Adolescents   191
12. Headaches in People Over Fifty   221
13. Less Common Headaches and Treatments   228
14. More Alternatives   246

Appendix A: Headache-Related
Organizations and Publications   267

Appendix B: Over-the-Counter Headache Medications   281

Appendix C: Medications
and What's in Them   291

Acknowledgments   317

Index   318

PREFACE

· · · · · · · ·

HEADACHE is an extremely common problem that affects tens of millions of people in the United States. As a headache specialist who suffers from migraines and daily headaches myself, I know firsthand the burden that headaches add to one's life.

In the past ten years, there has been a virtual revolution in the understanding and treatment of headaches. Yet headaches remain largely misunderstood by many physicians and patients alike and, in general, remain a poorly treated condition. Like asthma, shock, epilepsy, and many other medical problems once thought to be caused by stress or emotions, headache is a legitimate physiological medical condition, not a psychological one. People who get headaches do not bring them on themselves but rather have different levels of the brain chemical serotonin and a much greater reactivity of blood vessels about the head than others.

Despite tremendous strides in headache management, enormous amounts of time and money are wasted on useless diagnostic tests and treatments. As a result, headache sufferers, who have been unfairly blamed for their illness for far too long, become angry and frustrated, and many simply give up the search for effective headache therapy.

Many of the books currently available on headaches emphasize nonmedication techniques, which can be very useful but often only up to a point. These books give precious little information about the vast array of effective medications now available. Headache sufferers want to know more about their medications, and they should. Susan Lang and I felt there was a need for a book about the actions and side effects of the drugs that readers may take and the trial and error that is sometimes necessary to find the right medication at the right dose.

That's why this book places a strong emphasis on drug therapy. Nonmedication techniques are important, and *Headache Help* explores them fully. But for people who suffer severe headaches, these remedies often fall short, and medication becomes the primary key to treatment. Our aim is to provide as much reference material as possible so that lay readers can be better informed.

Headache sufferers should be commended for fighting through life with head pain. We hope the burgeoning knowledge about headaches will lead to more compassion for their suffering. With our new understanding of headaches as a physical problem, we can help the vast majority of patients tremendously with current therapies. If you or a loved one suffers from head pain, you should know all about the options; hence, we give you this book.

A caveat: Although we discuss many medications and treatments for headaches, this information is not meant to be prescriptive, suggestive, or a substitute for the medical advice of a physician. Only a doctor who understands your particular situation can make well-informed decisions about your treatment plan. Similarly, although we offer lists of common or first-line medication choices, there are always exceptions, and your doctor is best equipped to make this judgment.

Our intent is to provide information and education. In most cases, we could present only the common uses and side effects of medications. When you get a prescription, we still recommend that you ask your doctor or your pharmacist for details about possible side effects. *Physicians' Desk Reference* or the package insert also lists contraindications.

— Lawrence Robbins, M.D.
Northbrook, Illinois

· · · · · · · ·

SOME OF MY VIVID childhood memories are of my father's migraines. On bad days, he would retreat into his study, and the house became dark and gloomy. Although we four children tried to remember to stay quiet, we often forgot, and my mother would harshly scold us and banish us from the upstairs rooms. When would Daddy feel better and life resume its normal quality? Why did he have to get these things called migraines and disrupt our lives?

Since those days, my dad has "outgrown" his horrendous headaches, and we've emerged from the dark ages of headache treatments. But even the best treatments are useless if they are not sought out or adhered to. Information is empowering and is one of our most effective tools in our quest for better health and well-being. As a medical writer, my goal is to provide you with information so that you are not the passive recipient of a doctor's care, but an active, well-informed consumer.

To address those who may criticize Lawrence Robbins and me for focusing so heavily on medications: We do not minimize the power of mind-body techniques or of more natural therapies. Rather, we believe you should be fully informed of the full range of options. Only then can you properly weigh the risks and benefits of each potential therapy and weave your way through the maze of alternatives.

You deserve a pain-free life. We hope this book will help you achieve it.

— Susan S. Lang
Ithaca, New York

HEADACHE HELP

. . . .

1

· · · · · · · · ·

UNDERSTANDING THE
MODERN APPROACH

IF YOU'RE READING THIS BOOK, chances are you know the misery of headaches all too well. One moment life is normal, but the next your temples begin to ache and your forehead throbs. Soon your head is your worst enemy. The pounding, splitting pain of the headache overwhelms all else.

Contrary to what most people believe, you don't have to put up with it. If you get headaches frequently, don't despair; you can gain more control over them than you probably ever thought possible. Unfortunately, far too many people accept headaches as a fact of life. This attitude cheats you and your loved ones. Although headaches can't necessarily be cured, they can be controlled with certain lifestyle changes and, if needed, the wise and judicious use of modern medications.

Don't let headaches disrupt and complicate your life anymore. Take a stand. Learn what you can do to help yourself and your doctor to minimize the pain, agony, and frustration of headaches.

THE BAD NEWS

If you are one of the 45 to 50 million Americans who battle chronic headaches, you're probably not only miserable from the pain but guilty, depressed, and frustrated about missing work, disappointing loved ones, and giving up many of life's joys. You may fear that others view you as a malingerer, that your illness may jeopardize your job and future, and that maybe you are "crazy" and making yourself sick.

The truth is, headaches are a real physical illness and perhaps the most common medical condition plaguing human beings. They not only extort an exceedingly high price from individuals, but also from society. They are to blame for more than 157 million lost workdays a year in the United States at a price tag of some $20 billion in healthcare costs — including some 10 million office visits — and absenteeism.

The costly toll of headaches could be greatly reduced by better understanding how your lifestyle contributes to your headache pattern; how nondrug strategies, such as relaxation techniques, biofeedback, diet changes, and exercise, can make a significant impact; and how to use the right medication, chosen from a large and powerful arsenal. All you need is information, a willingness and commitment to try nondrug strategies, and in many cases, a trial-and-error approach to medication.

THE GOOD NEWS THAT FEW USE

Ironically, while a revolution has occurred in the headache field over the past ten years, most people who get headaches have failed to reap the benefits. Medical researchers understand the mechanisms of headache better than ever before. They have unlocked the mystery of how certain triggers set off headaches and how lifestyle changes can ward off many attacks. They have developed exquisitely specific headache medications that can quickly relieve or abort a potentially devastating headache. And for people who get frequent headaches, medical researchers now can provide low doses of certain medications to reduce sensitivity to headache triggers, thereby preventing many headaches from recurring.

Yet, tragically, although headache doctors now have the medical know-how to help more than 90 percent of headache sufferers, more than 70 percent of sufferers never even consult a doctor about their headaches.

WHY HEADACHES FAIL TO GET TREATED

Despite all the recent medical advances, many headache consumers passively endure the agony. Why? Because they mistakenly believe that little can be done to help them. Even worse, some people unwittingly aggravate their headaches by taking too many over-the-counter and prescription pain relievers and loading up on caffeine. Or they fail to give proven nondrug strategies, such as relaxation and other stress-reduction methods and exercise, a concerted try.

Others fail to seek medical help that could provide drugs that might change their lives. Of those who do consult doctors, many become quickly discouraged. Sometimes doctors are unaware of the latest treatments. Other times, however, consumers are given appropriate advice but are too suspicious of what may sound like a newfangled advance. Some patients think the doctor is fishing in the dark when the first medication doesn't work and a completely different one is prescribed. Although the doctor is following a very clear and reasonable strategy that often requires trial and error, the patient who is unaware of the rationale may become confused.

Still others may start a prescription medication but soon quit it, and they frequently never follow up with the doctor if it doesn't work or causes too many side effects. Some headache sufferers so fear the shift from a medication-free life to one suddenly cluttered with strange pills that they refuse to take their medicines consistently or correctly.

Instead, people spend billions of dollars trying all kinds of treatments on their own. Although some of these nondrug, natural approaches, especially relaxation and coping techniques, diet, and exercise, can and do prevent some headaches, many people still needlessly suffer because they either do not effectively institute the lifestyle changes required or because their headaches also require medication for relief.

HEADACHES ARE A REAL PHYSICAL ILLNESS

Before we get into the nitty-gritty details of treatment strategies, we need to get something straight: headaches are not psychological illnesses simply induced by stress but are genuine medical illnesses as legitimate as ulcers, diabetes, or heart disease. Stress may contribute to the muscle tension in the head or changes in the brain's blood vessels that cause pain, but researchers now know that headache mechanisms involve involuntary biochemical changes in the brain.

Those biochemical mechanisms in the brain seem to be inherited. In fact, migraine headaches, for example, are hereditary in up to 80 percent of sufferers. Researchers have evidence that the blood vessels in people with migraines are less sensitive and certain blood cells, called platelets, are less efficient than in nonsufferers in retaining serotonin, a neurotransmitter and chemical in the blood that not only helps reduce pain but constricts blood vessels. Its depletion is linked to migraine pain.

Other evidence for the physical basis of headaches stems from many studies that have revealed differences in the brain, arteries, and bloodstream in migraine patients. Mounting evidence from advanced brain scans shows similar differences in the brains of people with migraines as in those suffering anxiety. This finding is interesting because many people who have headaches are also anxious, and the two conditions seem closely linked in many people. It is also not coincidence that the drugs helpful for anxiety (such as the antidepressants) and headache (such as Imitrex) increase the level of serotonin. As scientists learn more about the physiology of migraines and anxiety, both conditions are increasingly being viewed as physical, genetic problems, just as many physical illnesses, once looked upon as "psychological" until the real causes were uncovered, are now known to be genetic and physiological.

As with many other conditions, the genetics of migraine are slowly being uncovered. A number of researchers have recently described the area of the "headache" gene, at least in certain families. So far, the research has focused on families with a certain kind of headache called a "hemiplegic" migraine, a rare type of migraine in which one side of the body becomes weak or numb for hours to days. Soon, researchers will know much more about the location of the migraine genes, which in turn could lead to better therapies or maybe even a "cure." Environment and stress play an important role, but headaches, like other physical illnesses such as asthma or diabetes, are the result of chemical and structural changes in the brain and bloodstream.

If you get chronic headaches, chances are you suffer from the bad luck of being born with a slightly different brain chemistry than most people, a sort of short circuit. Researchers strongly suspect that this different brain chemistry makes you more prone to painful dilated blood vessels in your head, and to the uncontrollable firing of the nerve cells in the transmission of pain signals. In other words, your brain chemistry makes you more likely to get headaches.

WHAT CAUSES AND TRIGGERS HEADACHES?

Although scientists still don't know the exact causes of headaches, many are convinced that the primary culprits are imbalances in the brain's chemicals and nerve pathways. The latest and most widely accepted theory is that the majority of headaches — namely tension headaches and migraines, which are thought to be on opposite ends of a spectrum — are caused by the depletion of the chemical serotonin, an important pain-reducing neurotransmitter (brain protein) that is involved in communication among nerve cells in the brain.

Serotonin plays an important role in regulating the diameter of blood vessels, that is, in constricting and expanding them, and, as we've said, it is the dilation of blood vessels which causes pain. Serotonin also stifles pain signals between nerve cells and influences sleep, anxiety, and mood (and is a factor in depression). Stress and other environmental factors are thought to influence levels of serotonin in the brain.

In normal cases, nerves that surround the blood vessels in the brain's protective covering, the meninges, release normal levels of neurotransmitters like serotonin, and no pain occurs. In headache cases, however, certain factors, such as stress or a particular food, trigger a chain of events in people born with troublesome serotonin regulation. Researchers think that first a wave of electrical activity spreads over the brain. Then the level of serotonin surges, and blood vessels around the brain constrict. Consequently, as the serotonin seeps into surrounding tissues, levels of the neurotransmitter fall in the brain. This decrease in serotonin causes the blood vessels to become inflamed and swollen, irritating surrounding nerves and perhaps the trigeminal nerve, a large and complicated nerve that extends to the blood vessels around the brain and into the face. The inflammation of the blood vessels and the irritation of nerves cause pain.

The serotonin pathways that play a vital role in migraines and probably tension headaches are the same pathways that influence depression, anxiety, and insomnia. Researchers have recently discovered that people with migraines in particular have a higher risk of depression, anxiety, and mild insomnia. While frequent headaches may cause a person to feel depressed or anxious, studies show that the increased risk of these conditions is independent of the headaches themselves. Migraine sufferers do, however, have much higher rates of panic attacks and moderately higher levels of chronic mild anxiety and nervousness (especially when the headaches are out of control), as well as more depression than people in the general population. Depression may aggravate preexisting headaches, but it does not cause headaches.

Serotonin attaches only to certain receptors in the brain, and different receptors may be associated with different conditions, such as headache, depression, and anxiety. Medications that fit on the serotonin receptors, and thereby mimic serotonin (such as sumatriptan), or influence serotonin levels (such as DHE, dihydroergotamine, and antidepressants) can help prevent and relieve both migraine and tension headaches. Other kinds of medications may help by either blocking the pain message, by constricting the swollen and inflamed blood vessels, or by stabilizing the blood vessels so they don't swell. Interestingly, many medications used for years because of their influence on blood vessels recently have been found to influence serotonin levels as well.

The muscles in the head may also contribute to headache pain by tightening up. But this occurrence is now believed to be the result of the headache mechanism rather than a cause of it. Nevertheless, once the muscles contract, they may contribute to the pain by releasing a toxic by-product, lactic acid, and reducing the amount of blood and oxygen that can get into the muscles.

Of course, not everyone gets chronic headaches. In fact, some people (the lucky ones) virtually never get a headache, regardless of what goes on in their lives, whether lack of sleep, illness, changes in hormones, or consumption of red wine. These people probably have the right chemical makeup in the brain to "protect" themselves against headaches. But if you are prone to headaches, probably because of some genetic or biochemical predisposition, serotonin imbalances probably occur more easily in you than in other people due to certain environmental, chemical, physical, and psychological factors. These triggers, which differ among individuals, include certain foods like chocolate and alcohol, bright lights, hunger, a changing sleep schedule, a hormonal shift, or psychological conditions like stress, anxiety, and depression. Sometimes even high altitudes, orgasm, and exercise may trigger headaches. Again, these factors aren't the causes of headaches; rather, they aggravate the biological condition that promotes the headaches. But by identifying which factors trigger your headaches and how to avoid them, you can learn how to relieve and prevent them.

TOO MUCH OF A GOOD THING: REBOUND HEADACHES

Ironically, people who suffer from chronic headaches all too often unwittingly make themselves sicker by overusing headache medications in their quest for relief. Too much caffeine — more than what is in three or four cups of coffee a day or in a more-than-twice-weekly dose of some pain relievers or decongestants — can seriously aggravate headaches. Even just two aspirin and some caffeine every day can turn occasional headaches into a chronic and severe headache problem while also making you less sensitive to many medications that might have helped you relieve or prevent the headache in the first place. Some 50 to 80 percent of all headache sufferers unknowingly fall victim to rebound headaches.

Unfortunately, it's all too easy to get caught in the rebound headache trap. Here's a typical scenario: You get a headache and find that a lot of caffeine or an analgesic, such as aspirin, ibuprofen (Motrin, Nuprin, Advil), acetaminophen (Tylenol), or a prescription vasoconstrictor (ergotamine) relieves it. Because it is so effective, you start taking it more freely. As your headaches escalate, so does your use of the caffeine or analgesic. As a result of the overuse, however, the substance becomes increasingly less effective — either because your blood vessels become somewhat immune to the substance or because the substance interferes with your body's ability to produce endorphins (natural morphinelike substances produced by your brain). As you become less sensitive to the caffeine or medication, you may try taking even more or try a new medication. The final result is that you end up with more frequent and severe headaches, and if you cut down, you still get headaches. In the case of caffeine, you may get weekend headaches if you drink far less coffee on Saturdays and Sundays than during the week.

So the very medications that can be most useful for headache relief can become your worst enemy. This syndrome is so common that some experts describe rebound headaches as an "unrecognized epidemic" in this country. In some cases, people must be hospitalized to go through the uncomfortable withdrawal process, which includes severe headaches. Ironically, withdrawal is all that is required in many cases to achieve significant relief from a chronic headache problem.

Because rebound headaches are so common among all kinds of

headache sufferers, learning how to balance your use of medications and caffeine can determine whether these substances will be among your best friends or ugly enemies.

HOW DOCTORS TREAT HEADACHES

If you suffer frequently from chronic headaches, your first goal is to do everything you can to avoid them by becoming well informed about foods and substances that may trigger them and how relaxation and coping skills, exercise, caffeine, and over-the-counter (OTC) pain relievers may help. If these approaches don't work, you should consult a doctor and ask about stronger, abortive medication to relieve a headache. Commonly, abortive medications, such as Midrin or Norgesic Forte, are used to prevent a mild or moderate headache from becoming severe. Other abortive medications, such as sumatriptan (Imitrex), can relieve a headache that has already become severe.

If you suffer from moderate to severe headaches more than three times a month and these episodes are severe enough to interfere with your family, job, or social life, then your doctor may recommend a preventive medication as well. Such drugs are not always completely effective, but they can minimize the frequency of headaches and the disruption to your life.

Many people don't want to take preventive medication because it means daily pill-popping. However, if you get frequent severe headaches that seriously impair your ability to get on with life's routines, your doctor may suggest switching from abortive medication each time you get a headache to preventive medication. Preventives are not only more benign than the abortives, but you end up taking less medication with preventives than if you just chase the pain with abortives. Also, abortive medications tend to be more addicting and have more side effects than preventive medication. We'll discuss guidelines for these strategies in subsequent chapters.

You must realize that trying a medication regimen is not a

permanent decision with lasting side effects. Medications may be used as temporary stopgaps to control a period when the headaches seem particularly overwhelming. After a spell, when the brain's misfirings seem to quiet down, you may go for months using only lifestyle techniques to prevent attacks. Then, for unpredictable reasons, if your biological mechanisms fire up again and set off another bad run of headaches, you may need abortive or preventive medications again for some time.

This is why becoming familiar with a headache doctor's medical approach is so important. By understanding the basic strategy — abortive versus preventive, as well as the options, risks, and benefits of each — you can make appropriate, well-informed decisions with your doctor. Then, using a rational, trial-and-error approach, you can decide together how to proceed if a medication is ineffective or has too many side effects.

TRIAL AND ERROR

Although lifestyle strategies that involve diet, exercise, relaxation, and the moderate use of caffeine and over-the-counter pain relievers (see Chapter 2) can help prevent headaches, when they fail to work as reliably as you'd hoped, prescription medications are the next resort. Only they can compensate for the differences in the brain chemistry or blood vessel changes that cause pain.

However, treating headaches is both an art and a science, and often the first try doesn't work. Each person is different: your headaches may be triggered by factors very different from someone else's and your response to medications is also unique. You need to work patiently in partnership with your doctor, who may need to experiment with doses, monitor you for side effects, and recommend several changes in medication before getting the right balance. Even after you find the right medication and correct doses, over time the medication may become less effective and your doctor may have to experiment again. At times this trial-and-error process may be frustrating, but try not to give up: The hope for a higher quality of life with fewer headaches should make up for the setbacks and stumbling blocks you may encounter along the way.

NONHEADACHE MEDICINES

You may wonder why your doctor would prescribe an antidepressant, anticonvulsant, or perhaps a medication used for high blood pressure or heart disease for your headaches. This approach isn't as odd as you may think. Certain medications commonly used to treat headaches are not always specifically approved or indicated by the Food and Drug Administration for this purpose. However, this practice is common. Medications often have several, sometimes a dozen, different effects. When drug companies develop and test a new medication — say, a drug with antidepressant, analgesic, sedative, and antiseizure effects — they focus on whatever property they think will be most marketable or profitable. In this case, they may focus their very costly research efforts on the drug's ability to prevent seizures. Once the drug is approved by the Food and Drug Administration as a safe and effective anticonvulsant, doctors may then decide to use it for an altogether different purpose.

Since swollen blood vessels are a primary cause of head pain, many medications used for headaches have a beneficial effect on blood vessels. The medications either influence serotonin, which in turn helps control blood vessel constriction and dilation; constrict swollen blood vessels directly; or help prevent blood vessels from swelling in the first place. Other medications, however, such as narcotics, help headaches by dulling the pain signal to the brain.

WHAT KIND OF HEADACHE DO YOU GET?

One of the first steps to understanding your head pain is to identify what kinds of headaches you get. Although there are about a dozen major types and more than sixty subtypes of headaches, the vast majority are either migraines or tension headaches, which most people will get from time to time, and to a lesser extent, cluster headaches. Many headaches that are believed to be common, such as sinus headaches and allergy headaches, are, in fact, quite uncommon. Many other types of headaches are actually very rare and are caused by serious disorders, such as brain tumors or meningitis, and can be identified by certain high-risk factors. See Chapter 2, "Symptoms to Take Seriously."

MIGRAINES
Migraines may afflict up to 25 million Americans, two-thirds of them women, many of whom get menstrual headaches as well. Migraines, which are usually inherited, are characterized by throbbing or aching pain, usually on one side of the head, and are often coupled with nausea and sometimes vomiting, visual disturbances, or dizziness. Numbness in an arm or area of the face may also occur. Some sufferers get so-called classic migraines with aura — they see colors, shimmering lights, or experience other kinds of visual changes. Without auras, the headaches are called common migraines.

TENSION OR MUSCLE-CONTRACTION HEADACHES
More than three-quarters of all headaches are tension headaches, previously called muscle-contraction headaches. Typically, as muscles tighten in your head and neck and blood vessels in your head expand, you feel a throbbing forehead pain, a dull pain on both sides of the head, or a sensation that your head is being squeezed, tightened, or pressed, as if in a vise. Although the name is "tension headache," stress and tension are not the major precipitating factors. Although we all get these headaches occasionally, some poor souls get them often, sometimes every day or every other day.

When these headaches are chronic, they are, like migraines, often the result of a genetically inherited, predetermined condition. Although the pain may stem partly from the muscles over the head contracting, researchers now believe that the root causes of tension headaches are the same as those of migraines: serotonin imbalances and blood vessel changes. When chronic, these headaches often need something stronger than over-the-counter pain relievers. And as with migraines, the use of OTC pain relievers can backfire and make these headaches worse.

CHARACTERISTICS OF THE MOST COMMON HEADACHES

Type of Headache	Onset	Pain	Who Gets Them	Pattern	Duration	Other Symptoms
MIGRAINES	Usually in childhood or by late twenties	Moderate to severe; usually one-sided; near an eye; pulsating or throbbing	70% are women	Several a month (from several weekly to several yearly)	Average: 4–8 hours; may last days	Visual disturbances; nausea/vomiting; dizziness; sensitivity to light and noise
TENSION	Any time	Mild to moderate; like a band or vise; across temples or head; usually not debilitating	Slightly more women than men	No periodicity	No clear beginning or end	Tightness in neck and shoulders
CLUSTER	In mid-life (between ages 20 and 45)	Excruciating; one-sided; sharp, like a knife	80% are men	Occur in clusters of time, usually weeks to months, once or twice a year	1/2 hour –1 hour	Flushed face; teary eye; stuffed or runny nose

CLUSTER HEADACHES

Afflicting about 1 out of 250 men and 1 out of 700 women, these agonizing headaches are among the most severe pains known to humankind. Their excruciating, debilitating pain, sometimes described as a red-hot iron being twisted around or through an eye or a temple, may last from fifteen minutes to three hours, sometimes longer. They're called cluster headaches because they occur in waves, usually lasting several weeks to several months, once or twice a year. Symptoms that commonly occur with clusters include a runny or stuffed nose, a teary or red eye, or a drooping eyelid on the same side as the pain.

LESS COMMON HEADACHES

POST-TRAUMATIC HEADACHES are the result of injuries from an accident (especially a car accident) in which the head or neck is involved.

SINUS HEADACHES are linked to colds, a runny nose, or hay fever and are not as common as you think. Most people who believe (or have been told) that they have sinus headaches (and get relief from decongestants) actually experience tension headaches or migraines (for which the decongestants may help because they contain caffeine) that are causing pain in the sinus region.

Except as a result of a sinus infection, most people don't get much of a headache from allergies or sinus congestion. However, migraines do engorge the sinus and create some stuffiness.

TMJ HEADACHES are also much rarer than most people believe. Although TMJ (temporomandibular joint syndrome) causes face pain and sometimes a headache, most chronic headaches in TMJ sufferers are actually migraines or chronic tension headaches. The TMJ may aggravate the preexisting migraine or tension headache problem.

EXERCISE AND SEXUAL HEADACHES may occur at any age, especially after exercise such as weightlifting, soccer in which the head is used, aerobics, jogging, diving, and sex. These headaches are usually benign (although they can be serious in rare cases) and often last only about twenty minutes, but sometimes as long as a day. Consult a physician if you experience exercise or sexual headaches.

ALLERGY HEADACHES are, in fact, rare. Most so-called allergy headaches are reactions, but not true allergic responses, to certain chemicals in foods that commonly trigger headaches. A mild headache may occur due to nasal or sinus congestion because of the allergies.

And as you'll see in later chapters, other factors, such as eyestrain, caffeine withdrawal, ear infections, an overactive thyroid, and dental problems, can also cause headaches. Certain medications can also give you a headache, such as nitrates (as in nitroglycerin) and hormones (estrogen or progesterone). Occasionally, people will get headaches from various medications for the heart, such as calcium blockers, nonsteroidal anti-inflammatories, medications for acid reflux or ulcers (such as Zantac), and from certain antidepressants (although, as we'll see, antidepressants can also help headaches), such as Prozac, Zoloft, Paxil, Celexa, Remeron, Serzone, and Effexor. Serious problems are rare, but you should rule them out by consulting a physician.

HOW HEADACHES AFFECT COUPLES AND FAMILIES

Although headaches are a legitimate illness, many families and coworkers tend to be less sympathetic to headaches than to other illnesses. Yet the effects of headaches may ripple through a family profoundly. When you get headaches, you may fail to fulfill your commitments as a spouse or parent because of the pain. When you suffer, your mate suffers too, driving you to the emergency room, making midnight dashes to the pharmacy, calling the doctor at all hours, preparing ice packs in the middle of the night, breaking plans, feeling emotionally and physically drained, bearing the burden of additional medical bills, coping with added child care and home responsibilities, trying to stay sympathetic to your moodiness during and after the headache, working with you regarding drug overuse or abuse, and so on, all due to your severe head pain.

You may have feelings of guilt, shame, anger, isolation, and inadequacy. Although you certainly are suffering, try to understand how your illness affects those around you as well. Chronic headaches are often a source of strife between partners. Some mates don't understand that the pain is the result of an inherited physical illness that is no more psychological than any other illness. Others fear that their partners take too much headache medication; although this may sometimes be true, it often is not. Yet it may appear to be a problem to a partner who doesn't understand why there are so many pill bottles in the medicine chest. Many headache sufferers need an array of choices — not only a pain reliever and perhaps a preventive medication, but also choices among these medications, depending on whether the headache strikes at night or during the day and whether they need to go to work or not. They may also need an antinausea medication. In addition, they may get new prescriptions when the current medication isn't strong enough but they keep the old prescription in case the new medication has too many side effects. The overwhelming majority of headache sufferers take medication simply for pain and nausea and do not abuse these medications for recreational use (although many do overuse them for pain).

Although headache sufferers are no more or less prone to addiction than others and simply wish to relieve their pain, family members may not understand and raise issues concerning medications and failed expectations. Your partner may need to suppress his or her own needs at times to care for you. This is tough when the headaches are chronic. Both of you need to try to understand each other's lot.

QUALITY OF LIFE

Medical researchers have made great strides in treating headache. A wide array of relaxation techniques and medications are available. The choices are wide, and finding the right one may take some time and trial and error. With proper treatment, you can learn how to gain control over your life, and enjoy relief and a restored high quality of life. We offer rational and reasonable strategies for a range of headache situations.

The road isn't straight, and often what seemed to be the right path becomes a dead end. You may have to backtrack, but it's worth it. After all, your life — and whether head pain will interfere with it or not — is what's at stake.

2

. . . .

HELPING YOURSELF

IF YOU GET frequent or severe headaches, you need to consult a physician. Nevertheless, you may want to know how to help yourself both with short-term techniques to get rid of a headache and long-term techniques to prevent future headaches.

Chances are, these self-help strategies won't always work, but if they can ward off some of your headaches so much the better. Before you consider self-help methods, however, you should understand that there may be something more serious going on than just a headache. If the following symptoms occur, consult a doctor as soon as possible.

SYMPTOMS TO TAKE SERIOUSLY

- The headaches get progressively worse over days or weeks.
- The headaches have started suddenly; you've never had them before (especially important if you're over fifty).
- The headache comes on suddenly after coughing, straining, or exertion, which has never happened before.
- You experience changes in memory, personality, behavior, or level of consciousness (that is, you become confused).
- You experience changes in vision or in your ability to walk, general weakness, numbness, or loss of senses.
- Your headache is associated with pain in the eye or ear.
- Your headache causes confusion or loss of consciousness.
- Your headaches are persistent, when previously you've never really had headaches.

- Your headaches interfere with your ability to function normally at work or in social situations.
- Your headaches are different from other headaches you've previously experienced.
- You have a stiff neck with a fever or a rash, or you experience a seizure.
- You have an unexplained fever or breathing problems, as well as the headache.
- There is a sudden or dramatic change in the severity of your headaches. If you get a very sudden and excruciating headache unlike any you've ever had, consult a doctor immediately.
- You get a headache after a head injury or accident, or after a sore throat or respiratory infection.
- You have a constant headache with no relief.

Assuming your physician rules out the possibility of a serious illness, here is a summary of the general guidelines for self-help methods to control headaches, which we'll examine in detail in this chapter.

HOW TO GET RID OF A HEADACHE: PRACTICAL STRATEGIES

- Practice a relaxation exercise.
- Drink something with caffeine, such as cola or coffee, or take a caffeine tablet.
- Try aspirin, ibuprofen (Motrin, Advil), or acetaminophen but not more than twice a week. The sooner you take it, the better.
- Apply reusable ice packs to the painful area.
- Try to sleep in a dark and quiet room.

RELAXATION AND DEEP-BREATHING EXERCISES

Far too many people discount the value of relaxation and deep-breathing exercises. Although considered totally unconventional just twenty years ago, these techniques have been successful in the East for centuries, and Western scientists have recently become more convinced of their powerful and beneficial physiological and psychological effects. They are now more widely accepted than ever before and are used in hospitals and clinics throughout the country as effective, legitimate, no-risk techniques.

If your pain is still somewhat mild, before reaching for a pill try just twenty to thirty seconds of a relaxation exercise, especially deep breathing and imagery techniques.

Relaxation in this context does not mean putting your feet up and reading the newspaper or watching TV. Rather, it is a technique to induce deep physical relaxation that reduces the body's response to stress by quieting both the mind and body. Physiologically, it can relieve pain by lowering your blood pressure, breathing rate, and pulse; reducing muscle tension and muscle spasms in your head and neck; increasing blood flow; and even stimulating brain waves associated with peace and tranquillity. Psychologically, these techniques help reduce distress, anxiety, and depression and promote a greater sense of calm, all of which can reduce pain.

Deep relaxation can also help change your perception and experience of pain and your response to it. By learning how to reduce the ill effects of stress, including its contribution to headaches, you gain a greater sense of control and mastery over your response to the stress. That control may also boost your hope and optimism and make you less conscious of your pain.

Many studies have shown the beneficial effects of relaxation and deep-breathing exercises. For example, during painful procedures, such as bone marrow transplants, when people practice relaxation methods, they have significantly lower pain ratings and pulse rates than when they take a tranquilizer or are distracted by videos. At Duke University, it has been shown that relaxation can help relieve lower back pain. And at the State University of New York at Albany, relaxation has been shown to help directly with chronic headache. Nausea and vomiting, which sometimes occur with migraines and headache medications, can also be significantly relieved with relaxation methods.

Unfortunately, although more doctors are now convinced of relaxation's beneficial effects, many people are unwilling to learn or to stick with these methods for very long. Some people resent being asked to try these techniques, believing they are mere mental tricks that minimize the legitimacy of their pain and suffering. Others feel silly or have no faith that they can help.

Yet if you acknowledge that pain escalates when you're upset, then you can understand how the opposite can be true: pain can be soothed when you're more relaxed. Also, because these techniques are safe, noninvasive, and have no risk of side effects, trying them can't hurt.

A few cautionary notes, however, are in order. These exercises are skills and as such they must be learned, practiced, and mastered. They cannot be adopted passively. They will be most effective for mild pain and can often avert the need to take an over-the-counter analgesic. Don't be discouraged if they don't seem to help on the first try. It may take up to two weeks to feel comfortable with these skills and to produce a beneficial effect.

PROMOTING RELAXATION

Various methods are commonly used to achieve deep relaxation, or what Dr. Herbert Benson has called the "relaxation response." These techniques include breathing exercises, physical exercise, visualization, autogenic training, progressive muscle relaxation, and biofeedback. Different people prefer different techniques. Use the one that helps you most easily achieve a sense of inner calm and peace. If you are able and willing to use your imagination with confidence, you will achieve the best results.

At first, try these techniques in a quiet location, sitting or lying down in a comfortable position with your eyes closed. Listening to soothing background music may further help promote a sense of calm. Once you become used to these exercises, you may be able to do some of them at work or even while driving (with your eyes open, of course).

CONTROLLED BREATHING OR MEDITATION Focus all your attention on your breathing for at least twenty to thirty seconds. Optimally, breathe deeply, slowly, and rhythmically, through your nose, deep in the back of the throat so you can actually hear your breathing. Hold the breaths for several seconds and exhale very slowly, completely emptying your lungs. Try tensing different muscles when you inhale and relax them when you exhale. Start with the toes and feet, and work your way up to your head. Some trainers suggest that upon exhaling you say a calming word or mantra to yourself (such as "relax," "peace," "beauty," or "love").

EXERCISE Any aerobic exercise, such as walking, biking, taking an exercise class, swimming, or playing tennis for at least thirty minutes, five times a week, can make a significant impact in preventing headaches. Regular aerobic exercise not only promotes the physiological relaxation response but boosts the production of endorphins (as does laughter and being in love), morphinelike chemicals that the brain produces. Endorphins give you a sense of well-being, raising your pain threshold as well as stimulating circulation, which bathes tissues in more oxygen and flushes out the body's toxins more quickly. Exercise may also be important in countering the effects of taking pain relievers frequently, as some researchers believe that frequent use of these medications may impair the brain's ability to produce endorphins. In addition to all its other benefits, exercise has also been shown to reduce stress, depression, and anxiety, which, in turn, can raise your pain threshold.

HEADACHE HELP TIP: BITS OF EXERCISE

You don't have to jog or go to an aerobics class for an hour a day to help your headaches. Exercising for little chunks of time — ten to twenty minutes — can make a difference. No matter how busy you are, you can fit exercise into your life if you think about it this way. First thing in the morning, consider walking for ten or fifteen minutes or using a treadmill. Ideally, you should aim for twenty to thirty minutes on average, but ten or fifteen minutes will do.

VISUALIZATION This technique can be added to the deep-breathing exercises. Visualization, also known as imagery, involves conjuring up a pleasant picture, imagining that you are in a beautiful garden, for instance, feeling soothed and relaxed. Visualization may also involve using your mind to imagine that physical changes are occurring. Pretend, for instance, that a magic wand is passing over your painful swollen blood vessels and causing them to constrict.

Many studies have found that there is more to these techniques than just taking your mind temporarily off the pain. By concentrating on pleasant scenes or magic wands that produce change, you can actually stimulate the same parts of the brain that are activated when you are experiencing the tranquil scene in reality, producing beneficial physiological changes that help promote relief for mild to moderate pain.

VISUALIZATION EXERCISE TO PROMOTE RELAXATION

Get as comfortable as possible and close your eyes.

You are on a tropical beach, and warm, soothing breezes are flowing over you. Imagine that you are floating dreamily on a raft in crystal-clear turquoise water. Feel the sun warming your body as the raft gently rocks up and down.

Imagine that the heat of the sun is warming your fingertips, your arms, your toes, your legs; it is bathing your painful forehead in its healing light.

Feel the bobbing motion and try to feel as weightless as possible.

Breathe slowly and deeply. Soon you are floating higher and higher, up to a large, beautiful cloud, drifting through the sky.

Imagine only calmness, warmth, and peace.

Other images to try are a crackling fireplace or a cool expanse of luxurious lawn.

Rather than focusing on relaxation only, you can also use a similar exercise directly on a painful area.

VISUALIZATION EXERCISE FOR PAIN RELIEF

Breathe slowly, deeply, and evenly. In your mind's eye, imagine that a magic wand is coursing over your head, bathing it in healing energy. As you inhale, pretend that you are bringing in warm goodness and healing energy. Hold your incoming breath as long as possible, and during that time imagine that you are squeezing and tightening the painful blood vessels in your head. Then imagine that the blood is flowing from your head, where all this pressure is, to your fingertips. As you exhale, imagine that pain, tension, and poisons are flushed out with your breaths.

AUTOGENIC TRAINING This technique is relatively simple. Repeat self-affirming statements involving warmth, heaviness, and calmness. By repeating the statements over and over, you lull yourself into a sense of calm and tranquillity, thereby promoting the relaxation response. At the same time, you may be able to warm your hands and feet if they tend to get cold (as they often do with migraines).

EXERCISE FOR AUTOGENIC TRAINING

In a dark room, close your eyes and get as comfortable as possible.

Repeat each phrase four or five times. For example: "My forehead feels heavy and warm, very heavy and warm. My forehead is getting even heavier and warmer. My forehead is sinking, sinking down into the pillow."

As you repeat your phrases, conjure up an image, as you

would in the visualization exercise, of a scene that brings warmth and pleasure. Repeat the phrases, each time substituting a different part of the head for "forehead" (eyes, sinuses, temples, top of the head, and so on), all the while breathing deeply and slowly. Your goal is to put your mind and body into a relaxed trance.

PROGRESSIVE RELAXATION TRAINING PRT involves tensing a part of the body, such as the hands or legs, for ten seconds, then releasing it from the tension. You squeeze each body part separately and sequentially, including every part you can think of, such as your forehead, eyes, and mouth, right down to your arms and fingers, feet and toes. After ten or fifteen minutes, you tense up the whole body and then allow it to go limp, releasing all tension.

Since many of us don't realize just how tense we really are and where we hold the tension in our bodies (neck or shoulder tension often contributes to headaches), PRT can help you identify the location of the tension and force you to relax. Several studies have shown that PRT can significantly reduce the severity and duration of nausea for cancer patients before chemotherapy (anticipatory nausea), and thus it may be useful to combat nausea linked to headaches.

SELF-HYPNOSIS Self-hypnosis integrates the techniques already described, namely deep breathing, visualization, and progressive relaxation training, to achieve the same deep relaxation response, and imagery to transform the pain sensations. The goal is to achieve a floating or drifting feeling, similar to your state just before falling asleep.

EXERCISE FOR SELF-HYPNOSIS

Sit or lie down in a comfortable position. Close your eyes. Relax your body as much as possible. Release any tension held until you feel limp and loose.

Then focus on your toes. Are they feeling limp? They should feel heavy. Be sure to release all tension. Then move to your feet. Do they feel limp and heavy?

Move up your leg, letting tension go each step of the way. Keep moving through your body, concentrating on each part and releasing all the tension in it. Tell yourself you need to let go completely and relax.

Breathe evenly and deeply, trying to focus your mind on the rhythm of the breathing, on the sense of feeling sleepy and deeply relaxed. Your entire body will soon feel heavy, limp, and loose. When you're done, open your eyes, slowly sit up, and then stand.

BIOFEEDBACK Biofeedback uses electronic equipment to monitor how successful you are with relaxation techniques to produce physiological changes. Biofeedback has been shown to help up to two-thirds of all headache sufferers who give it an earnest try. It is especially effective for teaching children and resistant adults that they can, in fact, exert some control over their body's response to stress.

By using painless electrodes on certain muscles and parts of the body, biofeedback electronically monitors body functions, such as breathing rate, blood circulation, heart rate, temperature, muscle tension, blood pressure, brain activity, and pulse. While being monitored, you practice the relaxation method of your choice and watch the instruments to see if you are actually producing physiological changes.

Temperature or thermal biofeedback can be very effective for migraines by helping you learn how to raise the temperature of your fingertips and achieve a relaxed state. The equipment lets you know how successful you are. Electromyographic biofeedback, on the other hand, which electronically monitors muscle activity, can sometimes be particularly useful for tension headaches by helping you learn how to release muscle tension.

Most pain clinics and hospitals have biofeedback equipment; however, sessions may be costly. Once you learn how to produce those physiological changes reliably, you will no longer need the machine to check you. For more information and referrals, see Appendix A.

MASSAGE, WARM BATHS, HOT TUBS, AND YOGA Combined with controlled breathing, any of these relaxation techniques may help you release tension and is worth a try to relieve mild headache pain.

Many audiotapes, available through bookstores and health magazines, can lead you through such meditations and relaxation exercises. Although not for everyone, such tapes, with their soothing background music or white noise (the sound of a night forest, for example), may help you drift into a trance, far from your painful headache. Many people feel refreshed, relaxed, and calm after listening. You may find it more useful to make your own tapes, with music and imagery you prefer.

CAFFEINE

In addition to a few moments of a relaxation exercise, you can help ward off a brewing and still somewhat mild migraine or tension headache by drinking a few cups of caffeinated tea, coffee, or a soft drink, particularly if you don't consume a lot of caffeine on headache-free days. Caffeine may help because it constricts dilated blood vessels, which often cause the pain. Caffeine may also raise serotonin levels, according to some studies. Because it is moderately effective in warding off headaches, caffeine is an ingredient in many over-the-counter pain relievers.

The best strategy for using caffeine is either to avoid caffeine completely on headache-free days or to keep your consumption down to one or two cups a day. Then if you feel a headache beginning, have a nice strong cup or two of your favorite caffeinated drink. The beneficial effect should last several hours; if you feel the headache creeping back again, you can have another cup.

If you don't want to have a caffeine drink, try a caffeine tablet that you can buy at the pharmacy. The rule of thumb is to take

CAFFEINE IN DRINKS, FOODS, AND MEDICATIONS

Foods and Drinks	Caffeine
Brewed coffee	75–125 mg per cup (drip is stronger than percolated)
Instant coffee	40 mg, but sometimes up to 150 mg, per cup
Decaffeinated coffee	2–5 mg per cup
Tea	30–50 mg per cup
Soft drink	40 mg per cup
Chocolate	1–15 mg per oz
Cocoa	Up to 50 mg per cup
Caffeine tablet (NoDoz, Tirend, and Vivarin; higher-strength tablets are available but not usually recommended.)	100 mg

Medications	Caffeine
Excedrin Extra-Strength	65 mg per dose
Anacin	32 mg per dose
Vanquish	33 mg per dose
Bromo Seltzer, Cope, Midol	30–33 mg per dose

(Appendix B lists the caffeine content of most over-the-counter medications used for headache.)

about fifty milligrams every three or four hours, as needed. Try to limit caffeine to two hundred milligrams, or, at most, three hundred milligrams per day. Your limit will depend on your sleep patterns, whether you suffer from anxiety, and if you are sensitive to rebound headaches. To see how much caffeine is present in different foods and medications, refer to the table opposite.

We can't stress enough that caffeine (and the pain relievers you'll read about in the next section) can also be one of your worst enemies. If you drink more than two cups of coffee or tea daily during the week but not on weekends, you're likely to get headaches from caffeine withdrawal. These rebound headaches flare up when the effect of the caffeine wears off after your body has grown accustomed to it.

If you're now consuming a lot of caffeine regularly, try to taper it to only one or two cups a day. Then you'll be able to use the caffeine to your advantage.

To enhance the pain-relieving effect of caffeine, you may also want to take one of the over-the-counter pain relievers discussed in the following section.

OVER-THE-COUNTER PAIN RELIEVERS

When you've truly tried relaxation exercise and caffeine to no avail, an over-the-counter pain reliever may be strong enough to help, especially if it is taken during the early stages of the headache. These pain relievers are combinations or single formulations of aspirin (or acetaminophen, Tylenol's main ingredient), with or without caffeine, and naproxen and ibuprofen, nonsteroidal anti-inflammatory drugs (NSAIDs). For the majority of people who get headaches, these medications are all they need.

But again, we must warn you about the risk of rebound headaches from taking these medications too often. Some people develop rebound headaches with as few as two or three of these pain relievers a day; others may not experience rebounds until they are consuming six or eight tablets a day. Nevertheless, it is important not to use these medications daily, but to restrict them to no more than twice a week. If you feel the need to use them more often, you should consult a doctor. Also, be sure not to mix more than one kind in the same day.

The best over-the-counter pain reliever for you will largely depend on your ability to tolerate the strongest ones. If nausea is a problem, you're well advised to avoid products with aspirin and the nonsteroidal anti-inflammatories. The medications in the following list appear in order of effectiveness, from most to least. Keep in mind that the stronger formulations are also more likely to cause side effects, particularly stomach or gastrointestinal irritation.

THE MOST USEFUL OVER-THE-COUNTER PAIN RELIEVERS FOR HEADACHES

1. EXCEDRIN EXTRA-STRENGTH, EXCEDRIN MIGRAINE, OR COMPARABLE PRODUCTS (ANODYNOS, BC POWDER, BC TABLETS, BUFFETS II, COPE, DURADYNE, MIDOL, PRESALIN, S-A-C TABLETS, SALATIN, SALETO, SUPAC, TRIGESIC, TRI-PAIN, VANQUISH)
Excedrin Extra-Strength and Excedrin Migraine contain acetaminophen (250 mg), aspirin (250 mg), and more caffeine (65 mg) than Anacin, which usually makes these medications more effective but also more likely to lead to caffeine rebound headaches when medication is stopped. (Excedrin Migraine has been approved by the FDA for treating mild to moderate migraines — the first over-the-counter medication to receive this approval.)

TYPICAL DOSE: One or two tablets every three hours as needed. To prevent rebound headaches or kidney damage, use cautiously, no more than an average of two tablets a day, fourteen tablets per week, or thirty tablets a month. If more is needed, see your doctor about taking preventive medication.

SIDE EFFECTS: The caffeine may trigger anxiety and the aspirin may trigger nausea. Less common side effects include stomach pain and heartburn. Long-term or high doses can cause liver or kidney problems and stomach bleeding.

2. NAPROXEN (ALEVE)

Naproxen, which has been a prescription medication for many years, is now available as an over-the-counter medication. It is a very effective and nonsedating medication. Coffee or a caffeine tablet may enhance its effectiveness. The prescription versions (Anaprox, Naprosyn) contain more milligrams of naproxen and are therefore stronger.

TYPICAL DOSE: One tablet (220 mg) with food or Tums or Rolaids. Total daily dose is three tablets, with eight to twelve hours between doses.

SIDE EFFECTS: Nausea and stomach upset, especially among people older than forty. With long-term daily use, liver, kidney, and gastrointestinal problems are a concern.

3. IBUPROFEN (ADVIL, HALTRAN, MEDIPREN, MIDOL 200, MOTRIN, NUPRIN, RUFEN, TRENDAR)

An inexpensive nonsteroidal anti-inflammatory (NSAID), ibuprofen is often helpful for tension and migraine headaches and reasonably well tolerated. Adding caffeine by drinking a cup of coffee or taking a caffeine pill can make the medication even more effective.

TYPICAL DOSE: From 200 (typical pill) to 800 mg every three to four hours as needed. Total dose should not exceed 2,400 mg per day, and if ibuprofen is used daily, blood tests should be taken to monitor potential liver or kidney irritation. Take with food or antacid.

SIDE EFFECTS: Commonly causes gastrointestinal upset. If you need more than an average of two pills per day, your doctor will probably recommend preventive medication.

4. ASPIRIN-FREE EXCEDRIN

Because it contains caffeine and acetaminophen only (no aspirin), it is not considered an NSAID. Without the aspirin, though, it tends to be less effective than Excedrin Extra-Strength. The lack of aspirin, however, makes it a good choice for people who tend toward ulcers, stomach upset, or excessive nausea.

TYPICAL DOSE: One or two pills every three or four hours.

SIDE EFFECTS: Seldom produces problems other than anxiety or insomnia from the caffeine.

5. ASPIRIN

Aspirin is extremely helpful in many cases and more effective than acetaminophen, but it also carries a greater risk of side effects. Avoid it during pregnancy or with gastritis or ulcer disease. It is available in many forms, including buffered, or coated, tablets.

TYPICAL DOSE: 325 to 650 mg every four hours as needed. Take with an antacid to minimize gastrointestinal irritation.

SIDE EFFECTS: Can irritate and cause bleeding of the gastrointestinal tract, thins blood and therefore prolongs bleeding time if you cut yourself, increases likelihood of bruising if you fall or bang yourself, and can cause reversible liver damage. Kidney irritation can occur with prolonged use of high doses.

6. ANACIN

Because it has less caffeine (32 mg) than Excedrin Extra-Strength, it is less effective but less likely to cause side effects or rebound headaches. It does contain plenty of aspirin: 400 mg in regular Anacin and 500 mg in Anacin Maximum-Strength.

TYPICAL DOSE: One or two tablets every three to four hours as needed. Take with food or an antacid.

SIDE EFFECTS: Because Anacin does not contain acetaminophen, it carries less risk of damage to kidneys or liver; its high level of aspirin, however, increases the risk of gastrointestinal irritation.

7. ACETAMINOPHEN

Acetaminophen is much less effective but better tolerated than aspirin or aspirin-containing products. It can be useful, however, for milder headaches, with minimal side effects, and may be used during pregnancy, with children, and with gastritis or ulcer disease.

Available in suppositories, tablets (regular and chewable), wafers, capsules, an elixir, a liquid, and as effervescent granules with sodium bicarbonate (Bromo Seltzer).

TYPICAL DOSE: One or two extra-strength tablets, 500 mg or 650 mg each, every three or four hours, limited to six pills per day. Do not exceed 4 g (4,000 mg) on any given day. If more than 1,500 mg is taken daily, rebound headaches may occur and preventive medication should be considered.

SIDE EFFECTS: If used excessively (5 to 8 g per day, over weeks), acetaminophen may damage the kidneys, liver, and heart.

8. KETOPROFEN (ORUDISKT)
This is a low-dose (12.5 mg) anti-inflammatory; the usual dose is two to four tablets every six hours, as needed. As with the other NSAIDs, stomach (gastrointestinal) side effects are common.

COLD AND HEAT

Reusable ice packs or wrapped ice is probably the most consistently effective nondrug therapy for headache. Ice packs help the pain by reducing swollen blood vessels. Be sure that the ice doesn't touch the skin directly but is wrapped with a layer of paper towel or a similar covering. Migraine Ice™ is a convenient method of using cold therapy.

Besides applying cold to the painful area, try placing it on the back of the neck, the top of the head, the forehead, temples, and so on. The earlier you use an ice pack to treat your headache, the better.

Heat (a very warm heating pad or a hot, wet washcloth) may be particularly useful during a headache to foster relaxation, increase blood flow, and relax your muscles.

Experiment to find out what feels good.

A COOL, DARK ROOM

Very often, simply taking a nap can give the brain an opportunity to get back to normal. Resting in the dark also helps because you may be particularly sensitive to light during a headache.

KEEPING A CALENDAR

So far, we've talked about ways to cope with a headache on the day it occurs. However, there are several strategies you can use to improve your headache situation in the long run. One of the most effective long-term strategies is to keep a headache worksheet, like the one shown here, for at least two months if you get frequent headaches. If you end up going to see a doctor, this will be an extremely valuable tool for assessment.

HEADACHE CALENDAR

Date	Trigger	Severity 1–10	Medication	How Well Did It Work?

If you are menstruating, mark the dates of your menstrual cycles on the calendar.

When filling in the "Trigger" column, consider the following list of triggers; they are listed in order of their importance and frequency among headache sufferers:

1. Stress
2. Weather changes
3. Hormonal changes: menstrual or premenstrual, birth control pills, pregnancy, menopause
4. Missed meal
5. Exposure to bright lights (particularly fluorescent or sun)
6. Lack of sleep
7. Foods eaten within twenty-four hours (check the list in Chapter 6)
8. Exposure to cigarette smoke
9. Exposure to perfumes or other odors
10. Letdown after stress
11. Too much sleep
12. Exercise or exertion
13. Seasonal change
14. Medications: oral contraceptives, etcetera.
15. Eyestrain
16. Travel by air, rail, car, bus

In the "Severity" column, enter a ranking from 1 to 10 using the following key:

1	3	5	8	10
none	mild	moderate	severe	excruciating

PSYCHOTHERAPY AND STRESS MANAGEMENT

Although headaches are not psychological illnesses, there is little doubt that stress and anxiety can trigger the headache mechanisms that otherwise may have lain dormant and can turn a mild headache into a more severe one. Psychotherapy and stress management can teach coping skills to reduce stress. Hundreds of studies in the past decade have consistently acknowledged the power of an effective coping personality and an optimistic outlook on health. Learning how to cope and bounce back from a setback rather than imagining that it is a catastrophe really can reduce the negative effects of stress on your body and may even help you live a healthier and longer life.

ENHANCING COPING SKILLS

When you change your mind, you change your life. By changing negative attitudes and automatic, self-defeating thoughts, you can diminish stress and anxiety. You can learn to monitor negative or unproductive thoughts or behaviors and learn how to respond differently. For example, you may exaggerate a situation or imagine potential catastrophes. Thinking these thoughts makes you feel anxious, depressed, or out of control. Imagining the worst makes it difficult to concentrate on productive ways of dealing with the problem.

Learning to focus on the brighter side rather than the worst-case scenario can help you view the circumstances in perspective and prevent stress from building up.

You may want to read one of the excellent self-help books on cognitive therapy (such as *Feeling Good: The New Mood Therapy* by David D. Burns, M.D., and *Learned Optimism: How to Change Your Mind and Your Life* by Martin E. Seligman, Ph.D.) or consider working in short-term therapy with a cognitive, behavioral, or task-centered psychotherapist. These approaches, which challenge the way you think about things, can help you diminish your daily level of stress and therefore reduce the likelihood of triggering the headache response.

EXERCISE IN COPING SKILLS

INSTEAD OF THINKING THE WORST:

"I think one of my awful and debilitating headaches is start-ing. That means I won't get that report in on time, which will affect my performance evaluation and could even jeopardize my job! If I lose my job, I'll never be able to pay the rent."

TRY A POSITIVE THOUGHT:

"My head is starting to hurt, but I know I can deal with it. I will practice my deep breathing and take a pain reliever. I just need to relax and I'm sure it will get better."

INSTEAD OF THINKING THE WORST:

"I'm all alone in this. Everyone thinks I'm a malingerer. No one is going to believe how awful I feel."

TRY A POSITIVE THOUGHT:

"Just because my daughter got angry that I couldn't go to her soccer game again, I can't jump to the conclusion that every-one's giving up on me."

INSTEAD OF THINKING THE WORST:

"This pain is killing me. I can't take it."

TRY A POSITIVE THOUGHT:

"This is a bad headache, but I must not panic. Relaxing will make it better. Remember to breathe deeply, in and out. Re-lax. The more I relax, the faster the pain will subside."

By consciously avoiding the worst-case scenario and looking at the more realistic side, you can shift your point of view from feel-ing helpless and hopeless to feeling more in control and more re-sourceful. An important coping skill to learn is replacing auto-matic, self-defeating assumptions and interpretations with a more positive point of view.

HEADACHE HELP TIP: HELP YOURSELF!

Here are some tips to prevent headaches:
- *Avoid stressful situations if you can.*
- *Try taking herbs that help you stay calm (kava kava).*
- *Wear sunglasses when you are outdoors.*
- *Eat small meals or snacks throughout the day.*
- *Keep to a regular sleep schedule.*
- *Try to avoid foods that you think trigger your headaches.*
- *Exercise at least fifteen minutes a day.*

PHYSICAL THERAPY AND CHIROPRACTIC THERAPY

In a recent poll of headache sufferers, physical therapy was identified as the most successful treatment after medications for helping
headaches. Often, several sessions of learning about posture, exercise, neck stretches, position of the body throughout the day, and
occupational hazards can be very worthwhile. For example, people who must bend their necks while on the phone all day often
get one-sided headaches and neck pain.

Many people with headaches also have neck pain and increased
muscle tension about the head. Chiropractic manipulation or
physical therapy can be very helpful to relieve neck tightness and
pain. Both of these treatments are discussed in more detail in
Chapter 14.

COPING WITH STOMACH PROBLEMS

If you get frequent headaches, you might also have frequent stomach problems. Gastritis (irritation of the lining of the stomach), ulcers (eroding of the stomach wall), and esophageal reflux (too
much acid backing up from the stomach into the esophagus, the
tube leading from the mouth to the stomach) are all common
problems that occur more frequently in people who get headaches.

Often stomach problems are caused by aspirin-containing products and other NSAIDs (anti-inflammatories). Stress can also produce an upset stomach.

If you are taking aspirin-containing products or over-the-counter NSAIDs and are experiencing stomach pains, talk to your pharmacist, or better yet, your doctor about buffered products that can protect your stomach. If you have reflux (heartburn), avoid big meals late in the day and try an extra pillow at night to keep your head higher than your chest. Being overweight may aggravate your problem, since excess weight adds pressure from the stomach to the esophagus. Also, avoid coffee and, to a lesser extent, tea and carbonated drinks. Although caffeine should be limited to 200 mg per day or less, caffeine does not directly irritate the gastrointestinal (GI) tract; the coffee itself does that. Also, see if avoiding spicy foods and chocolate helps.

For stomach medications, most people rely on the H2 blockers. Over-the-counter products, including Tagamet (cimetidine), Zantac (ranitidine), Pepcid, and Axid, which is available by prescription, can settle an upset stomach. Tagamet and Zantac are available in generic form; all of these are safe and usually effective.

The stronger "proton pump inhibitors" are more effective for reflux; these include Prilosec, Prevacid, and Aciphex, which are effective but expensive. Prilosec, in particular, is extremely effective for reflux. However, there is some concern that these medications are too effective in removing unwanted stomach acid, possibly leading to gastric cancer. Discuss these medications with your doctor before you take them.

Also, you need to check with your doctor not only to choose the right medication, but also to determine the reason for the gastrointestinal pain or upset. Many people have *H. pylori,* a kind of bacteria, in their stomach, which is easy to test for and treat with antibiotics. The treatments and drugs in this area of medicine have shown vast improvements since the days of Maalox, Mylanta, or Tums every two hours.

COPING WITH SLEEP PROBLEMS

If you get frequent headaches, chances are you often have sleep problems as well. That's because insomnia often coexists with headaches, probably because of inherited problems with serotonin regulation. If you do have sleep problems, here are some tips:

- Go to sleep only when sleepy.
- Get as much sleep as you need to feel refreshed and healthy, but not more. Curtailing the time in bed seems to solidify sleep; excessive time in bed seems to result in fragmented and shallow sleep.
- Set the alarm to get yourself up the same time every day to help you set your biological clock and circadian rhythms, which in turn can lead to a regular time of falling asleep in the evening.
- A steady, daily amount of exercise will probably deepen sleep; occasional exercise, however, does not necessarily improve sleep the following night.
- Occasional loud noises, such as aircraft flyovers or traffic, disturb sleep even in people who are not awakened by the noise and can't remember it in the morning. Sound-proofed bedrooms may help you if you must sleep near noise. Sound machines that put out "white noise" can drown out outside noise.
- Although excessively warm rooms disturb sleep, there's no evidence that an excessively cold room makes you sleep more soundly.
- Hunger can disturb your sleep; a light snack may improve your sleep.
- An occasional sleeping pill may help, but chronic use is ineffective in most insomniacs.
- Caffeine in the evening disturbs sleep even if you don't realize it.
- Alcohol helps tense people fall asleep more easily, but the sleep that follows is fragmented.
- If you get angry and frustrated because you can't sleep, don't keep trying to fall asleep. Get up and do something else.

Wait until you're really sleepy before returning to bed. If sleep doesn't come easily, get up and wait again. Repeat throughout the night as necessary.

- Use the bed only for sleeping and sex. Don't read, watch TV, or eat in bed.
- The chronic use of tobacco disturbs sleep.
- Don't nap during the day!
- Keep a night light on in the bathroom; bright lights will "wake up" your brain.
- Herbal supplements can be helpful (chamomile, valerian, kava kava, or a combination).

ACCEPTANCE

If you've suffered from headaches for years, it may help to accept the fact that you have this condition, and that there is no magical cure but that headaches can be managed and treated. Acceptance (but not resignation) will help relieve anxiety. By accepting your condition, you will no longer think "What have I done wrong? Can I find a cure? Why can't this just be cured?" Rather, your thoughts may be, "I have this condition; I need to keep informed, track my progress, and adjust my strategies. Don't give up. Headaches can be managed."

TO TREAT YOUR HEADACHES, KEEP THIS MOTTO IN MIND:

PATIENCE   PERSISTENCE   PERSEVERENCE

3

· · · · · · · ·

BEING A GOOD
HEALTH CONSUMER

ALTHOUGH the self-help techniques in the previous chapter are useful, they may not be powerful enough to control many of your headaches. If you get chronic or severe headaches, it is wise to discuss with a doctor how to manage them and to get prescriptions for medications to treat and prevent the more severe ones.

How effectively a doctor can help you control your headaches, however, will depend a great deal on your relationship with the physician. If communication is poor, even an effective strategy will be doomed to fail. In headache treatment, finding the right combination of medications and figuring out the correct dosages takes time and mutual cooperation. Choosing the right doctor is essential. This chapter will help you:

- Prepare for a doctor's visit.
- Determine what to look for in a doctor.
- Learn to be a good healthcare consumer.
- Learn how to best communicate your headache and associated problems.
- Learn how to help the doctor most effectively help you.

BRING YOUR HEADACHE CALENDAR
TO YOUR APPOINTMENT

As we discussed in Chapter 2, having a calendar that charts a series of previous headaches will be extremely useful to the doctor in analyzing what triggers your headaches and determining the type of headaches you get. If you haven't already done so, start a headache calendar as soon as you decide to see a doctor.

CHOOSING A DOCTOR

Ironically, many of us have learned to be good consumers of appliances or automobiles, investing much time, energy, and research comparing brands, energy uses, rebates, and so on, yet relatively few of us have learned to be good healthcare consumers.

For years, consumers took a passive role, subordinate and child-like, in their relationships with their doctor. The patient blindly accepted doctor's orders without question. Yet in this age of healthcare reform, the doctor-patient relationship is becoming more balanced. Consumers need to take more responsibility to inform themselves about their condition and to track their own case and medical history. Also, as a medical consumer, you now have more rights than ever — the right to understand treatment and alternatives fully, to assess the potential benefits and risks of each alternative, and to get a second opinion.

Many physicians will treat headaches, yet not all are up-to-date about the latest techniques in headache management. To assess a doctor's knowledge about treating headaches, you might:

- Ask a nurse in the practice what percent of the doctor's clientele are headache patients.
- Ask several local physicians to recommend the best headache specialist in the area.
- Ask the doctor how effective the treatment should be in relieving the pain.
- Ask about the doctor's strategy in treating your type of headache.
- Ask about the doctor's availability after you leave the office if you have problems with a medication.

Here are some warning signs that should alert you to the need to see another practitioner. The doctor:

- Treats your headaches purely as a psychological problem.
- Minimizes the importance of your pain or expresses any doubts about your pain.
- Discourages you from bringing or presenting a prepared list of questions.
- Has inappropriately low expectations for satisfactory relief.
- Does not fully discuss with you possible risks and side effects of new medication.
- Does not create an open environment in which you feel free to ask questions and express your needs, anger, and fears.
- Prescribes pain medication, such as Demerol or codeine, without trying a medication that aims to treat the root of the headache mechanism, such as serotonin imbalances and blood vessel changes.
- Does not encourage you to call if you experience unpleasant side effects or ineffective relief, or to schedule a follow-up visit in several weeks.

Although going to your family doctor for headache treatment may be adequate and appropriate for you, going directly to a neurologist who specializes in headaches, particularly if you think you need a comprehensive approach to your headache treatment, may save you a lot of money, time, and irritation in the long run.

If you fear that your doctor is less than fully knowledgeable about headaches, consider asking for a referral to a neurologist or a headache expert. You might say that you believe the doctor to be an outstanding internist, but every internist can't be expected to know the latest treatments for every condition. You might add that you'd like to take advantage of the recent strides in headache management, an emerging subspecialty, and state-of-the-art treatments that you understand are now available.

To ask for a second opinion, you might say, "I feel uncomfortable asking you this, but since this illness is so important to me, I need to obtain whatever information I can. I don't doubt your opinion. It's just that I need reassurance that this is the way to go. Do you have a colleague you might recommend for a consultation?"

Remember, you are the customer and need to be assertive about your own medical treatment. Free referrals can also be obtained through the headache associations listed in Appendix A.

HOW DOCTORS DO HEADACHE WORKUPS

When consulting with a doctor for headaches, be prepared to give a full medical history in as organized a way as possible. Chances are that the doctor will give you a form to fill out, similar to the "Headache Intake Assessment Form" at the end of this chapter. Note that this form includes the pain scale we've discussed earlier and potential headache triggers. Use your headache calendar to fill out such a form, or attach it to the form. Before you consult with the doctor, think about how you can best describe your pain. Consider the following:

- Is your pain one- or two-sided? Where about the head does it hurt (location of pain)?
- What's the typical pattern (frequency and duration of pain)? What's your headache history?
- Is there a time of day or month when your headaches are more likely to occur?
- What are your suspected triggers? Does exercise, exertion, fatigue, a certain food, or alcohol bring on or aggravate the attack?
- Do you have an aura (visual warning), tingling, or sense of numbness before a headache?
- Does anything make your headache worse or provide relief?
- Does your headache pattern change with your menstrual periods? Did it change during pregnancy?
- What medications do you take for headache? How frequently? What helps? What doesn't?
- What other medications do you take?

- What's your family's history insofar as headaches are concerned? (This question can be problematic, as many older people forget that they had headaches decades ago.)
- How do headaches affect your daily life? work? family? social life?
- What are your patterns concerning recreation? stress reduction? How do you experience stress (in your jaw, back, head, or elsewhere)?
- What are your past illnesses, allergies, experiences with different kinds of medications?

DESCRIBING PAIN

Be as specific as possible in describing the nature of the pain. One or more of the following may apply.

- piercing
- aching
- throbbing
- crushing
- boring
- burning
- pressing
- dull
- squeezing

Rate your pain severity as shown in Chapter 2, from 1 (very mild pain) to 10 (excruciating).

The doctor will listen to your heart, take your blood pressure, and test your nervous system through your reflexes, eye movements, and coordination. If you have a long history of migraine, tension, or cluster headache attacks that usually follow the same pattern, the doctor will be able to ascertain your problem and may not suggest a head scan, although such a test may be recommended for the legal protection of the doctor. A physician could be vulnerable, for example, if a chronic headache patient ever developed a brain tumor (which would be totally unrelated to these headaches) and the court challenged the decision not to obtain a test.

Nevertheless, in assessing your headaches, the doctor will need to eliminate the possibility of serious, though rare, physical problems as the root cause of the headaches, such as sinus disease, meningitis, glaucoma, brain tumor, bleeding in the brain, fluid on the brain, stroke, high blood pressure in the brain, and so on. The doctor may ask you seemingly strange cognitive questions, such as "Can you list the months of the year backward?" or other questions to test your memory, judgment, and ability to reason. These are not psychological evaluations; rather, they are used to evaluate whether any particular area of your brain is especially affected.

Although a full medical history and physical exam can eliminate many suspicions of more serious physical problems, the doctor may also prescribe one or more of the exams in the following list.

USEFUL TESTS FOR DIAGNOSING HEAD PAIN

- **Magnetic resonance imaging scan (MRI)**

A noninvasive procedure, the MRI allows the doctor to detect any serious causes of the migraines in the brain. While the MRI feels very claustrophobic and is expensive, it involves no radiation and is extremely sensitive in picking up any problems in the head.

- **Computerized axial tomography (CAT scan)**

Also called a brain scan. This procedure can provide information on the sinuses and potential tumors or strokes. An injection of contrast dye into the arm may be necessary.

- **Sinus x-ray**

Although an MRI or CAT scan provides more detailed information, a sinus x-ray is much less expensive.

- **Spinal tap**

Also called a lumbar puncture. This test is occasionally performed to assess certain nervous system conditions by evaluating the spinal fluid. It can cause a headache a few hours later. It is not necessary for most headache patients.

- **EYE PRESSURE TEST**

Also called intraocular pressure testing. An ophthalmologist does this procedure to rule out glaucoma.

- **BLOOD TESTS**

These tests can check for a variety of medical conditions, some of which may contribute to headaches, such as an abnormal thyroid.

- **ELECTROENCEPHALOGRAM (EEG)**

This procedure records the electrical patterns in the brain, which can provide valuable clues to the brain's functioning. This test is painless and safe and can be particularly helpful in assessing posttraumatic (concussion) headaches.

THE RESPONSIBLE PATIENT VERSUS THE "GOOD" PATIENT

You have a choice: you can be passive and just accept a doctor's recommendations even if they prove ineffective; ignore the doctor's advice and continue to suffer in silence; or discuss openly with the doctor your concerns, even though such a discussion may be uncomfortable, and ask for a change in treatment. Some people try to be "good" for fear that the doctor will otherwise view them as "difficult." They try not to complain, ask too many questions, or admit that a medication didn't work. Yet many treatment failures are beyond anyone's control, and most doctors expect them in some patients.

Being a good patient doesn't mean being an easy patient but a fully responsible adult working with the doctor as a partner and not undermining his or her recommendations. As a patient, you must work to understand the problems and complexities of your case, be knowledgeable about your condition and about the medication you are going to try, and understand the strategy that your doctor is using for your headache pattern.

Your doctor can be most effective when you either follow the recommendations or explain why you didn't. Yet only half of patients actually comply with their doctors' recommendations. Worse yet, some patients don't even tell their doctors they didn't comply. Little is gained if you go to your next appointment without having followed the strategy discussed at the previous meeting; all the time between the appointments is lost. Speak up or follow up by phone if you do not agree, do not understand, or have trouble following a recommendation. If you can't follow the doctor's recommendations, for whatever reason, call the office to make an alternate plan. Also, if you inconsistently or incorrectly take your medication, or take other headache-related medications at the same time without the doctor's knowledge, you can hamper treatment. The doctor can't know how to proceed properly if you didn't use the first-choice treatment rationally and correctly. Only if you communicate well can the doctor explain the treatment, or modify it, depending on your reaction.

HEADACHE HELP TIP: SWEETENING YOUR VISITS

If you're going to a doctor for your headaches, chances are that you will have frequent visits, as you and your doctor explore what works and doesn't work for you, to get prescriptions refilled, and get blood tests.

Personalize those visits — and get special attention from the staff — by bringing a treat, such as home-baked cookies, bagels and cream cheese, pastries from a local bakery, or a bag of candy. Not only does the treat lighten up the atmosphere at the doctor's office, but you will make friends with the office staff and become a person instead of a name.

You might also do the same for your doctor: A Cornell University psychologist found that physicians make better decisions when they're in a good mood, and that a little bag of candy or other token gift was all that it took to induce pleasant feelings. That positive effect can influence how your doctor solves problems creatively and makes decisions more efficiently.

You need to tell the doctor about all medications and drugs that you are taking, including over-the-counter and illegal ones.

Keep track in list form of what you've tried and what happened and keep a list of other medications you take (and the dosages) for other conditions. Bring this information to each appointment. Be sure to keep the doctor informed about other medical problems you may have.

ON BEING A GOOD HEALTH CONSUMER

Although the doctor is responsible for making proper assessments and recommendations, it is more important than ever that consumers take an active role in their own healthcare. To help prevent mistakes, track your own medical care. The doctor may, for example, prescribe a medication that could have an ill effect on an ulcer condition. Perhaps you had a problem with an ulcer some ten years ago; that information may not be on the front page of the medical chart. It's important for you to find out all you can about any new medication your doctor prescribes for you. Take responsibility by reviewing the drug information in this book or in reference books, such as the *Physicians' Desk Reference*. Standard reference books on medications, available in most public libraries, list contraindications or conditions to watch out for with each medication. Be responsible for bringing a concern from your medical history to the doctor's attention if it seems appropriate.

Also, the doctor may change the medication or dose for you over the telephone and neglect to make a notation of the change on your chart. Such mistakes happen. Doctors may also get sick or go on vacation, leaving a substitute who is unfamiliar with your case. If you can clearly convey the vital information the doctor needs, it will prove extremely helpful.

HEADACHE HELP TIP: SCHEDULING APPOINTMENTS

Consider scheduling your appointments for the first time slot in the morning or in the afternoon. By being first, you generally will not have to wait. If that's not possible, call the office before you leave for your appointment to find out if the doctor is running late. That can save you a lot of frustration — and time!

ACCEPTING ONLY SATISFACTORY RELIEF

It is your responsibility to follow up with your physician if you experience ill effects from medications and need to deviate from what the doctor prescribed. Don't give up if you come to a few dead ends. These are to be expected. Nevertheless, it's reasonable to expect a medication to improve your headache situation from 50 to 90 percent.

HEADACHE INTAKE ASSESSMENT FORM

Name:_____

Age: _____ Sex: M F

Marital Status: _____

Name of Spouse: _____

Name(s) and age(s) of children:

_____

_____

_____

_____

Education:_____

_____

Occupation:_____

Spouse's occupation:_____

Does anyone in your family have headaches? ___

Have they had moderate-to-severe headaches in
the past? _____

How often do you have a moderate-to-severe
headache? _____

How long do the severe headaches last? ___ Hours
___ One day ___ Two days
___ Three to several days

On a scale of 1 to 10, with 10 being the worst,
how severe are the headaches?

   1   2   3   4   5   6   7   8   9   10
       Mild   Moderate   Severe

How old were you when you started having
headaches? _____

Do you have some type of headache every day?

_____

How much do these daily headaches bother you?
   ___ Mildly   ___ Moderately   ___ Severely

Where does the pain hurt on the daily headaches?

_____

Where does the pain hurt on the severe
headaches? _____

What kind of pain is it?

Sharp ___ Pounding ___ Aching ___

Other: _____

Does your eye tear on the painful side of your head? _____

Have the headaches been much worse in the last few months? _____

Have the headaches been much worse in the last year? _____

Do you frequently have nausea with these headaches? _____ Does it bother you? _____

Do you have any visual problems, such as flashing lights or sprinkles of light, or do you lose your vision to one side with a headache? _____

For women only:

Are the headaches much worse before or during the menstrual period? _____

Are you on any birth control pill or hormone? _____

Does stress play a role in the headaches?

_____

Circle any of the following factors that play a role in your headaches or in producing an occasional headache:

Stress   Exercise

Weather changes   Missing a meal

Foods   Cigarette odor

Bright sunlight   Perfume odor

Relief from stress   Different seasons

Undersleeping   Summer

Oversleeping   Fall

Hormonal changes,   Winter

  such as menstrual cycle   Spring

Exertion   Sexual activity

Do you have very cold feet and hands in the winter? _____

Have you had a CAT scan for the headaches? _____
  If so, when? _____

Have you had an MRI for the headaches? _____

   If so, when? _____

Have you had blood tests in the past year? _____

   Were they normal? _____

Have you had any biofeedback or relaxation
training for headaches? _____

   If so, has it helped? _____

Which doctors/headache doctors, if any, have you
seen for headaches?

_____

_____

_____

_____

_____

_____

_____

List all medications
you have taken
for headaches,
including
over-the-counter   How much
ones and herbs   did it help?   Side effects?

_____   _____   _____

_____   _____   _____

_____   _____   _____

_____   _____   _____

_____   _____   _____

_____   _____   _____

_____   _____   _____

_____   _____   _____

_____   _____   _____

_____   _____   _____

4

. . . .

RECOGNIZING MIGRAINES

THE TECHNIQUES we've described thus far are most appropriate for preventing mild headaches or for keeping mild headaches from turning into severe ones. But for a chronic migraine sufferer, these techniques may fall short. A better understanding of migraines and migraine treatment will be essential for you to learn how to improve your quality of life.

Migraines can be devastating, with their sweeps of pain that can wipe out your ability to function and to think. Some 12 percent of us — about 18 percent of American women and 7 percent of men — are stricken at one time or another. Responsible for up to $15 billion in costs of absenteeism and billions more in diminished productivity and healthcare costs, migraines disrupt the lives of millions of Americans. Yet, to a great extent, these headaches remain underdiagnosed and undertreated.

In fact, according to a 1999 study sponsored by the National Headache Foundation, barely over half (53 percent) of people who suffer from migraines have ever been diagnosed by a doctor as having migraine headaches. Even more distressing is that only about one-third (34 percent) of migraine sufferers have ever consulted a doctor specifically about their severe headaches. Yet, three-quarters of migraine sufferers who have been treated appropriately report that the treatment has made a "dramatic improvement" in their quality of life.

WHO GETS MIGRAINES?

Most people who get migraines are probably born with a predisposition to them, which has been passed down from one generation to the next. At least four out of five migraine sufferers can identify a family connection, more than the sufferers of any other type of headache. Whether a person with an inherited predisposition actually gets frequent migraines depends on whether certain triggers (foods, bright lights, and so on, as explained in Chapter 6) aggravate his or her system enough to reach a threshold that sets off the migraine mechanisms.

Women are the most likely victims: they get migraines three times more often than men, probably because of all the hormonal changes they undergo.

Although migraines can strike at any age, most who are afflicted have well-defined migraines by their late teens and twenties, and then some get daily or almost daily tension headaches with occasional migraines later in middle age. These are called "transformed migraines" and add weight to the theory that migraines and tension headaches are part of the same headache spectrum. Some researchers believe that transformed migraines may actually be rebound headaches that develop from daily or almost daily use of over-the-counter medications, which turn sporadic headaches into frequent ones.

Occasionally, migraines and other kinds of headaches do begin in one's fifties and sixties. If this is your experience, be sure to consult a physician because headaches can be a symptom of certain medical conditions that become more common with advancing age, such as certain brain disorders, arthritis, heart or kidney disease, high blood pressure, anemia, spine disorders, and respiratory illnesses. Although the chances are that the headaches do not stem from one of these problems, they should be excluded as possible causes.

One popular myth is that well-educated and wealthy people get more migraines. The truth is, these people just go to doctors more often. Lower-income women, in fact, have the highest risk of migraines, perhaps because they endure more day-to-day stress trying to make ends meet. Stress, we'll see time and again, is a powerful trigger in setting off migraines and other types of headaches.

YOU ARE NOT ALONE

If you get migraines, not only do you join more than 20 million live Americans, but some pretty famous dead people, too. Famous migraine sufferers have included Julius Caesar, Saint Paul, Thomas Jefferson, Frederic Chopin, Charles Darwin, Tolstoy, and Sigmund Freud. Supposedly, Lewis Carroll, who wrote Alice in Wonderland, *might have been writing about what he felt or saw during a migraine aura.*

Do people who get migraines have a certain stress-driven migraine personality? Some people think that a certain type of person — a perfectionist who is excessively critical of himself and others, and who gets angry but holds it in — is more prone to migraines. Yet most headache experts disagree. As we've said, migraines are inherited biochemical conditions or predispositions, much like asthma and heart disease, and not the result of a high-strung personality. The "gene" for migraines has been identified in several families.

WHAT ARE MIGRAINES?

Whether caused by a chromosomal defect or biochemical imbalances, migraines and their diagnoses are not clear-cut. Typically, you will get a diagnosis of migraines if you suffer from recurring moderate to severe headaches that are triggered by stress, certain foods, weather changes, smoke, hunger, fatigue, or other factors. More specifically, if you experience at least four of these features, the chances are that your headaches are migraines.

COMMON FEATURES OF MIGRAINES

- Recurrent: usually one to five times a month, but sometimes less. Last four to seventy-two hours, occasionally longer
- Triggered by a migraine-precipitating factor: stress, certain foods, weather changes, smoke, hunger, fatigue, and so on
- Sensitivity to light, regardless of head pain (Many sufferers wear sunglasses outside during all daylight hours.)
- Blurred vision
- Nausea or vomiting, which sometimes eases the head pain
- Sensitivity to noise
- Tenderness about the scalp, which may linger for hours or days after the headache pain is gone
- Early-morning onset (but may be anytime)
- Throbbing, pounding, aching, or pulsating pain, usually on one side of the face or skull and often behind an eye (though sometimes the pain moves)
- Cold hands and feet (not just when a migraine occurs) and occasionally a cold nose
- Prone to motion sickness (not just when a migraine occurs)
- Dizziness or lightheadedness
- Lethargy
- Fluid retention, with weight gain (Some people start retaining fluids before an attack and gain up to six pounds, but the weight gain is temporary.)
- Vertigo, occasional but potentially disabling, during an attack
- Anxiety
- A sensation of burning, prickling, tingling, numbness (paresthesia), often occurring in one hand or forearm, but may be felt in the face, around the jaw, or in both arms and legs
- Diarrhea, usually mild
- Visual disturbances or hallucinations (auras)
- Stuffy or runny nose

LESS COMMON FEATURES OF MIGRAINES

- Mild loss of ability to read, write, or even speak (aphasia)
- Confusion
- Fever, or moderate increase in body temperature
- Seizures (rare)
- Loss of muscular coordination (rare)
- Temporary paralysis (rare)

Differentiating a mild migraine from a moderate or severe tension headache can be very difficult. Yet, if the headache is recurring, with repeated attacks of throbbing or severe aching, the headache is usually defined as a migraine, whether or not there is nausea, visual disturbance, or sensitivity to light and noise.

People with a migraine often become pale and, less often, flush. During an attack, they may also feel too hot or too cold. Sometimes, migraine sufferers experience pupil dilation or contraction, or a teary eye on the same side of the head as the pain. These are symptoms of a cluster headache, yet people with migraines often experience such aspects of cluster headaches, including the sharp pain about one eye or temple.

AURAS

When your migraine begins, you may see brightly colored lines or dots, known as an aura, thought to be caused when blood vessels supplying the brain and surrounding areas suddenly narrow, thereby reducing the blood flow in these tissues. Regardless of whether you have auras or not, the recommended treatment generally is the same. About 20 percent of sufferers, more commonly men, experience visual auras before the attack. Many people experience these auras only once or twice in a lifetime. Usually, they last fifteen to twenty minutes and may be as troublesome as the pain of the migraine. Sometimes these symptoms occur without pain, more commonly in adults over fifty. If you experience these symptoms, be sure to check with a doctor to rule out other disorders, particularly a condition called transient ischemic attack. Blurred vision is common during migraines, but it is separate and distinct from an aura.

VISUAL DISTURBANCES THAT MAY OCCUR WITH MIGRAINES

- Flashes of light
- Spots, stars, lines that are often wavy, color splashes, and waves resembling heat waves
- Shimmering, sparkling, or flickering images
- Mild loss in vision, with unformed hallucinations
- Dark spot in one's vision, often crescent-shaped, usually with zigzags. There is often a shimmering, sparkling, or flickering light at the edges of the dark spot.
- Graying or whiteout
- Blurred vision

PHASES OF A MIGRAINE

Migraines often occur in several stages.

WARNING
From hours to even a day before the pain begins, you may sense subtle neurological changes that are manifested by fatigue, irritability, depression, or moodiness. You may crave certain foods, yawn repeatedly, retain fluids, become more sensitive to light or sound, and be less attentive. Called the prodrome, this phase occurs in about half of migraine sufferers. If you experience it, you can learn to recognize the early symptoms, predict an attack, and prepare.

AURA

Not everyone who gets migraines experiences this phase. Typically lasting less than an hour, the aura includes visual disturbances, and sometimes neurological ones: you may experience tingling or numbness on one side of the face or down one arm, difficulty speaking or remaining perfectly coordinated, or one of the less common features listed earlier in this chapter.

If you experience auras, your migraines are considered classic migraines; those without auras are called common migraines.

PAINFUL HEADACHE

Lasting four to seventy-two hours, this phase is characterized by moderate to severe pain, often accompanied by sharp "ice-pick jabs." Most people describe their pain as throbbing, pounding, or pulsating, although some people feel a severe ache. Other symptoms during this phase include lack of appetite, nausea, vomiting, sensitivity to light and sound, and muscle tenderness in the head and neck.

RESOLUTION

In this phase, which may or may not occur, the pain is gone but you feel completely washed out, depleted of energy or depressed, and some people may even vomit. Others, however, feel completely relieved and calm, even euphoric. Sometimes, sensations similar to the warning phase may return (changes in food habits, moodiness, and so on). In addition, your scalp may remain sensitive.

CAUSES OF MIGRAINES

As we stressed in Chapter 1, migraine is an inherited physical illness, just like diabetes or asthma. Scientists still aren't sure what causes migraines. For many years, researchers believed that blood vessel spasms in the face, neck, and head caused these headaches.

The theory was that the initial spasm, or tightening, reduced blood flow, which caused general discomfort and the auras; then the blood vessels became inflamed, which caused pain.

The current theory suggests that when a person's migraine triggers build up and exceed the threshold, normal neurological functioning is disrupted. If the person experiences an aura, it is thought to be the result of a "spreading depression" over the brain. This is an electromagnetic or metabolic change, which has been observed in animals. It occurs like a wave and affects neurons in the brain. Changes in the blood vessels are probably the result, not the cause, of these changes in the brain.

Whether or not the aura occurs, scientists believe that something (perhaps dropping levels of magnesium) causes the trigeminal nerve, a large nerve that branches into the face and jaw and sends signals from the brain throughout the skull, to release small proteins called peptides. The peptides cause the surrounding blood vessels to swell, which in turn irritate surrounding nerve fibers, causing them to pulse and fire inappropriately and send pain signals deep into the brain.

More and more scientists are becoming convinced that serotonin, an essential chemical involved in communication among nerve cells, plays a key role in triggering migraines. The effectiveness of sumatriptan supports this theory. The medication works by binding to serotonin receptors, preventing nerve fibers from releasing their peptides, thereby quieting down the activity of the nerves and stifling their firings.

GENERAL MIGRAINE STRATEGY

Regardless of the biochemical causes of migraines, when you consult a doctor, the agenda typically will be:

- To determine whether you are getting rebound headaches from overdependence on caffeine or pain relievers and to help you get off them.
- To help you identify possible triggers, including specific foods.

- To be sure you understand the role of relaxation techniques, exercise, the use and overuse of caffeine and over-the-counter medications, and potential triggers.
- To give you an effective abortive medication, one that prevents a mild headache from worsening. These drugs work best if you have consistent warning signs even a half hour before the migraine actually starts raging. Abortive medications work either by preventing blood vessel inflammation, constricting blood vessels, blocking nerve cell pain signals, or changing the brain's blood chemistry.
- In some cases, to arm you with medication that can relieve disturbing side effects of a migraine, such as nausea or vomiting, and severe pain. These medications are pain relievers (some potentially addictive and, if misused, likely to cause rebound headaches) and antinausea medications.
- To find a daily preventive medication (one that is **not** potentially addictive) if you need abortive medication too frequently.
- To use a trial-and-error approach. The more you understand this strategy, the better you can help the doctor help you.

In other words, once it's clear that you are not experiencing rebound headaches or drug dependence, the doctor will try to prescribe medication to relieve your pain and other symptoms, with the goal of minimal medication and side effects.

Don't get frustrated if you and your doctor don't get it right the first time. Although you may feel like a guinea pig or that the doctor is stabbing in the dark, he or she is actually using a systematic trial-and-error approach. If you understand that approach, you will be able to make the treatment work most effectively and efficiently.

5

· · · · · · · ·

TREATING MIGRAINES
IN PROGRESS

IF YOU START getting a migraine, try to manage it with the techniques we describe in Chapter 2. In summary, these techniques include doing a relaxation exercise, having a caffeine drink or tablet, using an over-the-counter (OTC) pain reliever, applying ice packs, and napping in a dark room. When these techniques do not work, your doctor will probably prescribe an abortive medication, that is, a medicine used to relieve a headache in progress.

In discussing prescription medications, we'll separate them into "first-line" and "second-line." First-line medications are the first choices doctors turn to for various reasons. Through a process of trial and error, they will then try other ("second-line") options if the first-line medications can't be tolerated (produce side effects), or if they are ineffective or inappropriate because of other medical conditions.

QUICK REFERENCE GUIDE: FIRST-LINE MEDICATIONS FOR TREATING MIGRAINES IN PROGRESS

1. **TRIPTANS (IMITREX, MAXALT, AMERGE, ZOMIG, RELPAX)**
   Very effective, no drowsiness or stomach problems, but not for people with major heart disease risk factors.
2. **NONSTEROIDAL ANTI-INFLAMMATORIES (NSAIDs) (NAPROXEN, IBUPROFEN, KETOPROFEN, CELEBREX, VIOXX)**
   Nonsedating, but stomach upset is common.

> **3. ASPIRIN AND CAFFEINE (EXCEDRIN EXTRA-STRENGTH, EXCEDRIN MIGRAINE, ANACIN, BC HEADACHE POWDERS, VANQUISH)**
>   Stomach upset fairly common.
> **4. MIGRANAL NASAL SPRAY**
>   Safer than standard ergotamines; stuffy nose and nausea fairly common.
> **5. MIDRIN**
>   Mild enough for children, but fatigue is common.
> **6. BUTALBITAL COMPOUNDS (FIORINAL, FIORICET, ESGIC, ESGIC PLUS, PHRENILIN)**
>   Contain a barbiturate sedative so are potentially addictive; commonly cause fatigue, lightheadedness, and nausea.

When a migraine comes on and over-the-counter tactics don't work, most doctors will prescribe a triptan (Imitrex, Amerge, Maxalt, Zomig, Relpax), NSAIDs, aspirin and caffeine compounds, Migranal Nasal Spray, Midrin, or one of the butalbital compounds (Fiorinal, Esgic). Ideally, a migraine medication would not simply mask your pain; it would stop the migraine in its tracks in the brain. Triptans and these other medications leave you alert and able to function. While pain medicine may help to relieve the pain itself, your quality of life is much better with pure migraine medications, such as Imitrex and the other triptans.

Unfortunately, some doctors use heavy-duty narcotic medications just to treat the pain, rather than using a first-line medication to influence the headache mechanism itself. The narcotics are powerful medications that in most cases should be used as a last resort. If migraines strike frequently, well-informed doctors will use a preventive treatment (see Chapter 6) in addition to an abortive one.

Choosing a first-line abortive medication, or deciding to jump to a second-line abortive, depends on:

- Your risk factors for heart disease.
- Your age. Some medications, as you'll see, should be avoided by certain age groups.
- Whether nausea occurs. If so, avoid aspirin and the non-steroidal anti-inflammatories. Also, avoid those products if you have an ulcer or gastritis.
- Whether you need to work and function at optimal levels. If so, you should probably avoid the sedating medications.
- Your experience with each medication. Often one medication won't work for you but a similar one will. For someone else, the opposite may be true.

Although many of the medications described in this and subsequent chapters have not received specific approval from the Food and Drug Administration (FDA) for migraine use, they are considered reasonable, appropriate, and common treatments for headaches. Consult your doctor before taking any of the following medications.

As with other descriptions of medications in this book, the information that follows is a guideline and is in no way prescriptive.

Here are some details on first-line abortive medications. The over-the-counter medications are listed in their order of consideration; refer to Chapter 2 for more information about them.

Please note: For most headache medications, particularly the "as-needed abortives," the generics do not work as well as the brand names. Although generics contain the same compounds as brand names, their binders and other substances are often less effective. As a result, brand-name medications may be absorbed into the bloodstream more thoroughly.

FIRST-LINE MEDICATIONS
FOR ABORTING MIGRAINES

1. TRIPTANS

The triptans have revolutionized the treatment of migraines. Doctors now prescribe fewer preventive medications than in the past because the abortive triptans are more effective. These medications, which include Imitrex, Maxalt, Amerge, Zomig, and Relpax, ease headache pain without causing excessive drowsiness, nausea or stomach problems, addiction, or difficulty in thinking. These medications work by raising the level of serotonin in the brain and thereby reducing dilation of the surrounding blood vessels. They often lift the headache away, rather than simply covering over the pain. That's why many people describe triptan as a "miracle medicine."

Triptans are effective for about 65 percent of migraine sufferers. However, people who have more than minimal risk factors for hardening of the arteries should generally avoid them. These risk factors include: poorly controlled high blood pressure, strong family history of coronary artery disease or heart attacks, diabetes, high cholesterol, smoking, male gender, or older age ranges. In general, doctors use these medications with caution, although they have been deemed safe under most circumstances. They should not, however, be used if you're pregnant or nursing.

So far, six triptans have been approved, and more are on the way. Like NSAIDs, these medications have many similarities but also important differences. Amerge, for example, tends to have fewer side effects, while Imitrex gives more relief to more people; Maxalt tablets work faster than other triptan tablets, while Imitrex Nasal Spray or injections are the fastest. So even though these medications are quite similar in safety, if you don't tolerate one of them, you can try another and have a pretty good chance of finding one that is appropriate.

It may be worthwhile to try two or even three types of these medications before giving up on the triptans.

- ### SUMATRIPTAN (IMITREX)

Imitrex is the gold standard in migraine abortives. It was the first triptan developed and used, and it has been given to over 15 million people worldwide. It is available in nasal spray, injection, and tablet form, with tablets the most convenient. If you have severe nausea, however, you may prefer the nasal spray or injections. The nasal spray is slightly milder than the tablets but is quickly absorbed and works somewhat faster than the tablets. The injections are somewhat more difficult to use but faster-acting and more effective than virtually any migraine-abortive medication.

TYPICAL DOSE: One tablet (50 mg) every two to four hours as needed, four per day at most. Some people use 25 mg (half a 50 mg tablet or a 25-mg tablet), and some people use 100 mg at a time. While the average dose is 50 mg, doctors try giving just half a tablet the first time a person uses a triptan to see what the effect will be. This way, side effects, if any, will be minimal.

Imitrex Nasal Spray is available in 5-mg and 20-mg sizes. Each spray dose is for one-time use only. Most patients need the 20-mg spray. The usual dose is one spray every three to four hours, as needed, two per day at most. Imitrex Nasal Spray is usually considered about equal to the tablets, both in strength and efficacy. Side effects are similar with the tablets and the spray.

You should limit the nasal spray to two 20-mg sprays per day at most, separating them by at least two hours. Only one spray and two tablets at most should be used in a single day.

The nasal spray is easy to use, and its instruction sheet is easy to follow. Basically, you should keep your head in an upright position, close one nostril, insert the nozzle of the nasal spray into the open nostril, and press the blue plunger on the Imitrex. The nasal spray, of course, allows for much more convenient dosing than the injection. It is usually sold in a box containing six sprays. The spray is well tolerated but can leave a bad taste in the mouth. Keeping the head upright can help. Sucking on candy or drinking juice or pop may also help offset the bad taste.

The injectable form (subcutaneous) is the most effective migraine abortive for severe, fast-onset migraines. The usual dose is one injection every three to four hours, as needed, two in one day at the most. The injections can be used in the same day as the tablets or the nasal spray; one tablet is equal to one nasal spray, and approximately two tablets or two nasal sprays equal one injection. The usual limit is ten tablets per week, ten sprays per week, or five injections per week at most. Habitual use at this level is not recommended, however.

SIDE EFFECTS: Tightness in the muscles, particularly in the throat, chest, or jaw, may occur. If you experience more than mild chest heaviness or muscle tension in the chest muscles, you should probably discontinue using a triptan. Occasionally, a triptan is retried after a cardiac workup has been done. Serious heart side effects, though extremely rare, have been reported with Imitrex and the other triptans. Tingling in the fingers or toes, sedation, a rash, shortness of breath, or "spaciness" are also side effects linked to the triptans. These side effects tend to be short, usually lasting no more than one hour. Occasionally, however, side effects may last longer. Many people do not experience any side effects at all.

TRIPTANS WITH OTHER MEDICATIONS: The ergotamines should not be used in the same day, nor should one triptan be used in the same day as another triptan. Pain medications (Fiorinal, Vicodin, codeine) may be used in the same day or even at the same time as a triptan. Antiemetics (antinausea medications), such as Phenergan, Reglan, or Compazine, are safe with triptans.

- ### RIZATRIPTAN (MAXALT)

Maxalt is a well-tolerated triptan available either as a tablet to swallow or a dissolving tablet to put on your tongue. The dissolving tablet, Maxalt MLT, has a slight minty taste and does not require any water. Maxalt has a similar profile to Imitrex, with approximately the same effectiveness.

TYPICAL DOSE: One tablet, 10 mg, may be taken every three to four hours as needed, three in a day at most. You should limit the tablets to no more than ten tablets a week. Maxalt MLT tablets have the same instructions as the tablets you swallow. Maxalt can take anywhere from 20 minutes to two hours to help.

SIDE EFFECTS: Side effects are very similar to those of Imitrex. These include nausea, chest heaviness or pressure, pressure in the throat, shortness of breath, rash, tingling sensation, particularly in the fingers, heat sensation, tiredness, drowsiness, and dizziness. However, as with Imitrex, most of the side effects, should they occur, are brief. If they are more than mild, Maxalt should not be taken again. Caution is recommended for people who have more than minor risk factors for heart problems.

MAXALT AND OTHER MEDICATIONS: The same restrictions apply as to Imitrex. It should not be used in the same day as ergotamines or other triptans.

• **NARATRIPTAN (AMERGE)**

Amerge is very similar to Imitrex, but its effect lasts longer. It's considered the "kinder, gentler triptan." It takes longer to work, but tends to give relief all day. While Amerge is available in 1-mg and 2.5-mg strengths, the vast majority of people need 2.5 mg per dose. Amerge and other long-acting triptans are sometimes used in specific situations to prevent headaches (such as for menstrual migraines). Amerge is best for slower-onset, more moderate migraines. Imitrex, particularly the nasal spray or injections, may be a better choice for severe, fast-onset headaches with moderate to severe nausea.

TYPICAL DOSE: One tablet every three to four hours as needed, two in a day at most. Most people only need one tablet. The very first time you use Amerge, try a half tablet to see how you will react to it.

SIDE EFFECTS: The side effects are very similar to those of Imitrex and Maxalt, but Amerge is usually tolerated better. Amerge may be taken in the same day or even at the same time as pain medications (such as aspirin, ibuprofen, Fiorinal, Vicodin, Tylenol). However, do not use ergotamines (Cafergot pills or suppositories) or other triptans in the same day.

• **ZOLMITRIPTAN (ZOMIG)**

Zomig is another in the growing list of triptans. The usual dose is 5 mg every three to four hours, as needed, two per day at most. Zomig is also available in a 2.5-mg tablet. Zomig has the same general tolerability and efficacy profile as the others. Like the other triptans, Zomig may have short-lasting side effects.

- **ELETRIPTAN (RELPAX) AND FROVATRIPTAN**

  These are newer triptans, available in tablet form. More clinical experience is needed to determine what role these newer triptans will play.

2. NONSTEROIDAL ANTI-INFLAMMATORIES (NSAIDs)

These are very useful nonsedating medications if you don't become nauseated with a migraine. If one of these anti-inflammatories doesn't help, try another. It may be worthwhile to try two or even three types before you move to something else. If you're over age fifty, however, chances are your doctor will not recommend these drugs, because as you get older, you become more sensitive to these drugs' gastrointestinal side effects. A newer class of NSAIDs (Celebrex, Vioxx), however, has fewer gastrointestinal side effects.

The NSAIDs (naproxen, ibuprofen, ketoprofen — all available over the counter) are discussed in detail in Chapter 2. The typical doses and side effects listed there also apply to migraines.

- **NAPROXEN (ALEVE, NAPRELAN):**

  This OTC medication is a very effective, nonsedating medication, but unfortunately often causes stomach upset, especially in people over forty. It is particularly useful for menstrual migraines and is commonly used as a preventive medication (see Chapter 6). Aleve is available over the counter in 220-mg tablets. Prescription naproxen is available in a variety of doses, from 250 mg to 550 mg. Taking it with coffee or a caffeine tablet may enhance its effectiveness. Naprelan is an excellent, long-acting form of naproxen.

  TYPICAL DOSE: Two Aleve (440 mg total) with food to start. If you do not experience any significant nausea, repeat in one hour, and then at three- or four-hour intervals, taking six per day at most.

  SIDE EFFECTS: Nausea and stomach upset, especially among older people. With long-term daily use, liver, kidney, and gastrointestinal problems are a concern. Metoclopramide (Reglan), a medication for nausea, may help offset the side effects and increase the effectiveness of naproxen.

- **IBUPROFEN (AVAILABLE OVER THE COUNTER IN 200-MG TABLETS AS ADVIL, NUPRIN, MOTRIN)**

Ibuprofen is not as long-lasting as Aleve, but some people find it as or more effective. The usual dose is two or three tablets with food every three to four hours as needed, with the total dose not exceeding 2,400 mg per day. Adding caffeine, either by coffee or in pill form, often enhances its effectiveness. Stomach upset is fairly common.

- **KETOPROFEN (OrudisKT)**

This over-the-counter anti-inflammatory is available in 12.5-mg doses. The usual dose for a migraine is two or three tablets with food every three to four hours, as needed. Eight tablets per day is the maximum. As with ibuprofen and Aleve, stomach upset is relatively common. Taking it with caffeine may increase the effectiveness.

- **COX-2 INHIBITORS (VIOXX, CELEBREX)**

These newer anti-inflammatories are the first ones not to cause stomach upsets and ulcers as the other anti-inflammatories often do. So called because they block an enzyme called Cox-2 that triggers pain and inflammation, these drugs are popular for arthritis, menstrual pain, and other acute pain. They are being studied to determine their effectiveness for headaches. Although Cox-2 inhibitors are deemed safe and are used by millions of people, one recent study raised questions about their safety in a very few older patients. Their safety, therefore, has not been definitively established.

If you take a Cox-2 inhibitor, do not take another anti-inflammatory such as Advil, aspirin, or Aleve. However, a Cox-2 inhibitor can be utilized with low-dose aspirin if you take aspirin for prevention of stroke or heart attacks. Tylenol is OK as well. People who have had reactions to sulfa antibiotics should not take Celebrex. Vioxx is particularly good because it is long acting and indicated for acute pain. The usual dose is 12.5 or 25 mg (tablets) every four hours, as needed, 50 mg in one day at most. If used daily, it should be limited to 25 mg per day.

3. ASPIRIN AND CAFFEINE (EXCEDRIN EXTRA-STRENGTH, EXCEDRIN MIGRAINE, ANACIN, BC HEADACHE POWDERS, VANQUISH)

Aspirin and caffeine are old standbys for migraine relief. As with the NSAIDs, though, they may trigger gastrointestinal upset. The addition of Reglan, a mild antinausea medication, may help offset nausea and increase effectiveness.

- **EXCEDRIN EXTRA-STRENGTH, EXCEDRIN MIGRAINE**
  Excedrin is excellent for mild to moderate headaches and usually is well tolerated. This is a very effective over-the-counter medication, but it can cause anxiety, nausea, and less often, stomach pain. Its 65 mg of caffeine is more than in most OTC pain relievers, which can help to relieve pain but can occasionally lead to anxiety. The usual dose is one or two tablets every three to four hours as needed. Excedrin has proven to be one of the best medications for mild to moderate migraines.

- **ASPIRIN-FREE EXCEDRIN**
  Although less effective than Excedrin that contains aspirin, this OTC drug does not cause stomach irritation, making it especially useful for people with ulcers or for those who often get nauseated. This is an extremely useful preparation but not quite as effective as Excedrin Migraine.

- **ANACIN**
  Anacin contains slightly more aspirin (400 mg) but less caffeine (32 mg) than Excedrin. For some people, Anacin is more effective than Excedrin, and vice versa. The usual dose is one or two tablets every three to four hours, as needed; six per day at most. Stomach upset or nausea is common because of the increased amount of aspirin. The lower dose of caffeine results in less anxiety and nervousness compared to other high-caffeine compounds.

- **BC HEADACHE POWDERS**
  These contain 650 mg aspirin and 32 mg caffeine along with salicylamide. Some patients do better with a powder because it may be absorbed more easily into the bloodstream. The increased amount of aspirin is helpful for headaches but can lead to more stomach upset and nausea.

- **VANQUISH**

Vanquish primarily contains aspirin, acetaminophen, and caffeine. The usual dose is one or two tablets every three to four hours as needed. As with the others, anxiety, nervousness, or stomach upset may occur.

4. MIGRANAL NASAL SPRAY

This is DHE (dihydroergotamine) nasal spray, available in pharmacies. While it is technically an ergotamine (see page 79), DHE is safer than the standard ergotamines, because it shrinks the veins more than the arteries. Since 1945, DHE has been associated with only a handful of serious side effects.

TYPICAL DOSE: One spray in each nostril, usually repeated in ten to twenty minutes. Two sprays in each nostril in a day at most.

SIDE EFFECTS: Stuffed nose and nausea may occur. A feeling of being hot or flushed in the head or muscle cramps occasionally occurs. While less effective than the triptans, Migranal Nasal Spray is generally a safe and well-tolerated migraine medication.

5. MIDRIN

Midrin has held up over the years as one of the best headache medications. A combination of a blood vessel constrictor (isometheptene mucate), a mild sedative with no addiction potential (dichloralphenazone), and acetaminophen, it is extremely effective and well tolerated. It can be prescribed for children as young as five and is safe with the elderly as well.

Although Midrin may cause fatigue, taking it with caffeine (either strong coffee or 50 to 100 mg of caffeine, as found in NoDoz) can counter this effect while at the same time enhancing the drug's overall effectiveness.

TYPICAL DOSE: One or two capsules when headache begins, then one capsule every hour as needed but no more than six per day or twenty per week.

The first time you try Midrin, take only one capsule because fatigue or lightheadedness may be overwhelming with two.

For children or others who have difficulty swallowing the large capsule, pull it apart and spread the contents in applesauce or yogurt. This method may also be used when only half a capsule is needed.

Generic Midrin is not as effective as brand-name.

SIDE EFFECTS: Generally well tolerated, but fatigue or mild stomach upset is common. Occasional lightheadedness. Can raise blood pressure so is used with great caution among those with high blood pressure.

6. BUTALBITAL COMPOUNDS

All these medications are potentially addicting because of the butalbital, a barbiturate sedative, but they are considered safe and effective when used sparingly. The generic forms may not be as effective as the brand names.

- ### FIORINAL

  This drug is the most effective of the butalbital compounds because it contains aspirin instead of acetaminophen; it also contains caffeine and butalbital. Many people experience a brief high or euphoria with the medication, however, and this effect can lead to addiction. It is important not to take it, therefore, to relieve stress and anxiety.

  TYPICAL DOSE: One or two pills every three hours as needed, but should not be taken more than two days a week; no more than forty pills per month. Occasionally, use of one or two on a daily basis is justified.

  SIDE EFFECTS: Fatigue, lightheadedness, nausea, and euphoria are relatively common. Anxiety or rebound headaches occur occasionally. When taken for anxiety or stress, may lead to abuse.

- ### FIORINAL WITH CODEINE, FIORICET WITH CODEINE

  Though more effective than Fiorinal in relieving a migraine, the codeine causes more side effects. A major concern of using this medication is its potential for abuse.

  TYPICAL DOSE: One capsule every three hours, or two every four hours, as needed.

SIDE EFFECTS: Fatigue, lightheadedness, and nausea are common. Many people can't tolerate the codeine; stomach upset or abdominal pain are fairly common.

- **FIORICET, ESGIC, AND ESGIC PLUS**

These medications are particularly useful if aspirin nauseates you because Fioricet, Esgic, and Esgic Plus contain acetaminophen instead (Esgic Plus contains additional acetaminophen). Otherwise, these drugs are similar to Fiorinal (in that they contain caffeine and butalbital). This substitution of acetaminophen for aspirin makes these medications less effective but also less troublesome, especially regarding nausea.

TYPICAL DOSE: One or two pills every three hours, as needed. Each Esgic Plus pill contains 500 mg acetaminophen; no one should consume more than 4 g (4,000 mg) daily.

SIDE EFFECTS: Fatigue and lightheadedness are most common; occasional nervousness; nausea is uncommon but may occur. To avoid addiction, these medications are usually not taken for daily headaches.

- **PHRENILIN**

Phrenilin is similar to Esgic but has no caffeine; it contains butalbital and acetaminophen. (Phrenilin Forte contains extra acetaminophen.) Although less effective than Fiorinal or Esgic, Phrenilin is useful for people who can't tolerate caffeine or aspirin or who take medication at night when they want to sleep. Many doctors recommend using Fiorinal or Esgic in the morning or afternoon and Phrenilin at night.

TYPICAL DOSE: One or two pills every three hours, as needed.

SIDE EFFECTS: Fatigue is most common because this medication has no caffeine to offset it. Occasional lightheadedness.

HEADACHE HELP TIP: WHEN TO GO FOR THE BRAND

Unfortunately, the generic medications for relieving headaches generally do not work as well as brand names. For ex-

ample, the butalbital medications, such as Fiorinal, Esgic, Fioricet, Phrenilin, Fiorinal or Fioricet with codeine, and Midrin, seem to do a better job than their generics (butalbital and duridren, respectively). The generics have to include the same ingredients, but the fillers don't have to be the same. Sometimes the brand name is just better.

ADDICTION VERSUS DEPENDENCE

Before going on to other medications, we should point out that addiction is different from dependence. *Dependence* on a medication is an expected effect of some drugs; it means that you need the medication to reduce pain or improve the quality of your life. People who are dependent on a medication will need to take it but do not constantly increase the dose. If they stop taking the medication, they may have to reduce the dose gradually, depending upon the drug.

Addiction, on the other hand, connotes a psychological craving for a drug. People who are addicted to a drug may constantly want to increase their dose, obsess about the medication, call the doctor's office or clinic frequently about the medication, often with phony stories about how the medication was lost or destroyed, go to multiple doctors for the medication, or call in phony prescriptions to the pharmacy without the doctor's consent.

The overwhelming majority of people who are prescribed pain medications do *not* become addicted. Dependence on the medicine is relatively common, but this is acceptable and to be expected with daily pain. Addiction, however, is not acceptable. Studies generally show that only one or two people out of one hundred who are prescribed pain medications actually become addicted. The reasons for addiction are many but include the fact that these medications may help anxiety and depression, and increase energy (at least for a short time). If you have an addictive personality or have had a problem with an addictive drug in the past, including alcohol, it is extremely important that you share this information with your physician. If you've had an addiction problem in the past, you may still use a narcotic for pain relief, but you should use narcotic medications judiciously and in very limited, controlled amounts.

SECOND-LINE MEDICATIONS
FOR ABORTING MIGRAINES

If the first-line medications are not appropriate for you or have proven ineffective, a doctor may recommend one of these second-line medications.

QUICK REFERENCE GUIDE: SECOND-LINE MEDICATIONS FOR TREATING MIGRAINES IN PROGRESS

When the first-line medications aren't appropriate or don't work for you, your doctor may choose one of these:

1. **ERGOTAMINES (CAFERGOT, ERGOMAR)**
Effective but often cause nausea, nervousness, dizziness, and sleeplessness.

2. **KETOROLAC INJECTIONS (TORADOL)**
An anti-inflammatory with no sedation or potential addiction effects; particularly good for people who tend to vomit with migraines.

3. **CORTICOSTEROIDS (DECADRON, PREDNISONE, DEPO-MEDROL)**
Very effective but can only be taken for brief periods; long-term use can lead to weight gain, adrenal gland suppression, and other problems.

4. **NARCOTICS (MILD: CODEINE, DARVON, VICODIN, VICOPROFEN, ULTRAM, AND OTHERS; STRONG: STADOL NASAL SPRAY, DEMEROL, METHADONE, PERCOCET, PERCODAN, OXYCONTIN, TYLOX, AND MORPHINE) AND SEDATIVES (VALIUM, KLONOPIN)**

The narcotics should be taken with antinausea medication. Sedatives can cause sedation and drowsiness. For many patients, these drugs can help.

5. DHE INJECTIONS

Very effective if you can give yourself injections, but nausea is common; not for people over sixty, or those with angina or poorly controlled high blood pressure.

1. ERGOTAMINES

These medications are often effective because they constrict blood vessels that have become abnormally dilated. But they often cause many side effects, including nausea and anxiety. If these medications are overused, the resulting rebound headaches can be severe. People over forty should use ergotamine with caution because this drug increases the risk of heart attack.

• **CAFERGOT PILLS**

These are among the most commonly used ergotamines because they may be taken orally and are thus more convenient than their suppository counterparts; they are, however, the least effective of this group. They must not be used more than one day in four to avoid the risk of rebound headaches.

TYPICAL DOSE: One or two pills when pain begins, repeating every half hour or hour; no more than five a day or ten a week. When used two days in a row, rebound headaches may result.

SIDE EFFECTS: Nausea with occasional vomiting is common. Nervousness, difficulty sleeping, and dizziness may occur. Less common are numbness, tingling, or muscle pain in the fingers or toes.

• **CAFERGOT SUPPOSITORIES**

Though less convenient than pills, these suppositories, which contain caffeine and ergotamine, are much more effective. They're usually not a good choice, however, if you tend to get diarrhea with your migraine.

TYPICAL DOSE: Starting with one-third to half a suppository, the dose may be adjusted up or down depending on the
patient's response. No more than two per day, one in four days,
or four per week is recommended.

SIDE EFFECTS: Same as for the Cafergot pills but with less
nausea.

- **CAFERGOT PB SUPPOSITORIES**

More effective with fewer side effects than suppositories without pentobarbital but not as widely available. A generic preparation is available, and certain pharmacists can prepare these
suppositories themselves. Cafergot PB Suppositories contain
caffeine, ergotamine, and pentobarbital, which can cause sedation but helps reduce nausea.

TYPICAL DOSE: Same as for the Cafergot Suppositories
without pentobarbital.

SIDE EFFECTS: Same as for the Cafergot Suppositories
without pentobarbital but significantly milder. Sedation, however, is more common with this preparation.

- **ERGOMAR**

This is a pure ergotamine (2 mg) with no caffeine. Limit the
dose to two in a day, one day out of four only. This drug produces less anxiety than Cafergot.

2. KETOROLAC (TORADOL)

Ketorolac is a moderately effective anti-inflammatory. It's a
good choice when you want to reduce risk of sedation or addiction or if you can't take medication orally because you tend
to vomit with your migraines. Like many other medications,
this drug is more effective when injected than when swallowed
in pill form. The injections are available in convenient, prefilled syringes, but the needle is large. Individual vials are now
available.

TYPICAL DOSE: When injected, 60 mg is a typical dose, which
may be repeated in an hour if needed. No more than 120 mg per
day, only once a week.

SIDE EFFECTS: Stomach upset or pain, occasional sedation.

Possible liver or kidney problems; people with any liver or kidney impairments should not take ketorolac; older people should use it very cautiously.

3. CORTICOSTEROIDS

Cortisone (either pill or injection) is one of the most effective medications for severe, prolonged migraines and menstrual migraines, but it can only be taken in small doses and for brief periods of time. Long-term use of cortisone can cause serious side effects, such as weight gain, adrenal gland suppression, and predisposition to fractures and liver failure.

Dexamethasone (Decadron) and prednisone are oral medications; Depo-Medrol is administered by injection.

TYPICAL DOSE: One tablet or a half, usually 20 mg prednisone or 4 mg Decadron, taken with food, and repeated every four to six hours as needed. No more than three tablets per month. None of the corticosteroids should be taken with NSAIDs, or gastrointestinal bleeding can occur.

When migraines are triggered by flying, a half or whole Decadron or prednisone pill should be taken a half hour before flight time. For altitude migraines, take one pill a half hour to an hour before your plane arrives in a high-altitude city or before you reach a high summit. Take another pill four hours later. The dose can be repeated for two days.

For severe, prolonged migraines, Depo-Medrol injections (40 to 80 mg) may help, but limit to once per two months at most.

SIDE EFFECTS: Possibly nausea, insomnia, stomach upset, nervousness, and facial flushing. Occasional weight gain or water retention. More rarely, fatigue or agitation.

4. NARCOTICS AND SEDATIVES

When triptans, DHE, ergotamine, ketorolac, or one of the corticosteroids doesn't help or causes too many side effects, a strong narcotic, usually given with an antinausea medication, may be the answer. Doctors may be somewhat more reluctant to use these medications because of their potential for nausea as well as for abuse that can lead to addiction. Typically, these medications can calm you and induce sleep. They are useful only for one to three days and shouldn't be used every day unless every other method for controlling daily headaches has failed. (See the section on addiction versus dependence earlier in this chapter.)

- **MILD NARCOTICS**

  The milder narcotics, or opioids, can be taken by mouth.

  - **ACETAMINOPHEN WITH CODEINE (TYLENOL 3, WITH 30 MG CODEINE, AND TYLENOL 4, WITH 60 MG CODEINE)** has no aspirin and therefore induces less nausea.
  - **ASPIRIN WITH CODEINE** contains aspirin (which is good for migraines) and codeine, but also tends to induce nausea.
  - **HYDROCODONE WITH ACETAMINOPHEN (VICODIN, ZYDONE, NORCO, AND LORCET)** is well tolerated for a narcotic medication. Zydone and Norco contain less acetaminophen.
  - **VICOPROFEN** contains 750 mg hydrocodone plus 200 mg ibuprofen. This is an effective combination but may lead to stomach upset. More effective than Vicodin.
    TYPICAL DOSE: One every four to six hours, as needed.
    SIDE EFFECTS: Nausea, sedation, addiction.
  - **PROPOXYPHENE (DARVON OR DARVOCET)** is sometimes helpful for migraine sufferers when the other mild narcotics aren't. As with many medications, each person responds differently.
    TYPICAL DOSE: One or two pills every three or four hours, as needed. Limit to six pills per day at most.
    SIDE EFFECTS: Nausea, sedation, addiction.
  - **TRAMADOL (ULTRAM)** is an excellent milder painkiller. Ultram has combined opioid and serotonin-level action; unfortunately, this drug *causes* headaches in some people while relieving headaches in others. Tramadol may cause nausea or fatigue, but is generally well tolerated. The usual dose is one or two tablets every four to six hours as needed. In rare cases, Ultram can be addictive but is less so than the other narcotics.

- **STRONG NARCOTICS**

  Sometimes these strong medications are the only ones that will help a severe migraine. No more than three or four tablets a day or ten pills a month for any of these medications is recommended. Injections offer better pain relief than tablets and may be administered with an antinausea medication.

- **BUTORPHANOL (STADOL)** nasal spray is a strong narcotic that is slightly different from the others. It is called a "mixed agonist/antagonist," which sets it into its own class. Stadol is convenient because it can be used if you feel nauseated. The usual dose is one spray in one nostril only, every four to six hours as needed. Side effects may be severe and include sedation, fatigue, and confusion. However, when used properly, Stadol has been a safe medication. It is habit-forming and should not be used for daily headaches except in rare circumstances.

- **MEPERIDINE (DEMEROL)** injections are more effective than tablets.

  TYPICAL DOSE: For oral meperidine, 50 to 100 mg every three to four hours, as needed; 50 to 125 mg per injection.

  SIDE EFFECTS: Nausea and drowsiness, sometimes constipation. Can be habit-forming if used often.

- **METHADONE (DOLOPHINE)** lasts longer than Demerol and carries less potential for nausea and addiction.

  TYPICAL DOSE: 5 or 10 mg per injection, every three to four hours, 20 mg per day at most.

  SIDE EFFECTS: Same as with meperidine.

- **OXYCODONE (PERCOCET, PERCODAN, TYLOX, OXYCONTIN)**

  TYPICAL DOSE: One tablet (5 mg oxycodone with aspirin or acetaminophen) every three to four hours. Injections are not available. Oxycontin is the slow-release, long-acting form.

  SIDE EFFECTS: Same as with meperidine.

- **MORPHINE**

  TYPICAL DOSE: For tablets, 15 mg every three to four hours, or 10-to-15-mg injections.

  SIDE EFFECTS: Same as with meperidine.

HEADACHE HELP TIP: FOR SOME PEOPLE, NARCOTICS MAY BE HELPFUL

Myths die hard. Until recently, few physicians considered narcotic medication appropriate for noncancer pain because of dangers of addiction. Recent studies have shown, however, that very few people who use opioids for pain become addicted. The American Pain Society and the American Academy of Pain Medicine both endorse opioid treatment for selected cases of chronic noncancer pain, such as severe headaches. Many doctors now understand that although some patients may need increasing doses for pain relief, that need is usually caused by intensifying pain. They also expect physical dependence with narcotic medication but distinguish that from addiction, which is a psychological craving. People who are dependent on opioids because of pain syndromes can be withdrawn gradually from the medication.

- **SEDATIVES**

Sedatives are always useful for severe migraine because sleep is a powerful weapon against headache.

  - **BENZODIAZEPINES**
    - **DIAZEPAM (VALIUM)**

    A sedative and a muscle relaxant, Valium may be less effective as a generic.

    TYPICAL DOSE: 5 or 10 mg every three or four hours if necessary but no more than 20 mg a day. Should not be used daily.

    SIDE EFFECTS: Sedation, disorientation, and euphoria; may increase depression if used frequently.

    - **CLONAZEPAM (KLONOPIN)**

    A somewhat stronger sedative than Valium, Klonopin is often used to induce sleep. It should not be used daily unless other means have not been helpful.

TYPICAL DOSE: 0.5 mg to 2 mg every three or four hours, as needed. No more than 4 mg a day.

SIDE EFFECTS: Drowsiness, sedation, and fatigue. Flu-like withdrawal symptoms may occur if medication is used for a long time and then suddenly stopped.

HEADACHE HELP TIP: PHARMACIST PREPARATIONS

Many pharmacists can prepare different forms of certain medications, which are not otherwise commercially available.

- **SUPPOSITORIES**
For patients too nauseated to take a pill. Many kinds of mixes are available, such as a pain reliever with an antinausea medication.

- **LOZENGES**
Particularly good for children who won't swallow pills but also useful for combining a pain reliever with an antinausea medication.

---

5. DHE (DIHYDROERGOTAMINE) INJECTIONS

DHE has been available for more than fifty years for relieving migraines. Before that, ergotamine tartrate, a similar medicine but one with more adverse effects, was used. In addition to constricting arterial blood vessels mildly, DHE probably works by also modulating serotonin. This medication is safe, well tolerated, and very effective, particularly if you are willing to give yourself an injection (it is not available in premeasured auto-injectors so you must draw the medication up into a syringe). It is not as effective as sumatriptan but lasts longer and carries no risk of rebound headaches. Recently, new ways of administering DHE have made it more practical. It can now be taken through an IV, injection, or as a nasal spray. Injections are still the best way to get quick headache relief, but the nasal spray is the easiest route and can be effective.

DHE is not a good choice for people who are pregnant, have

angina, poorly controlled high blood pressure, or poor circulation in their hands or feet, or are over age sixty.

TYPICAL DOSE: As an injection, 1 mg (one vial) is typical, but 0.5 to 1.5 mg is not uncommon. Although DHE does not cause rebound headaches, 5 mg in a week should be the limit. DHE may be used for two days in a row.

SIDE EFFECTS: Although there are many possible side effects, they are unlikely to last more than a day, and serious side effects are very rare. Most side effects last less than an hour.

Nausea is very common, so it's often a good idea to take anti-nausea medication (such as Reglan, Compazine, Tigan, or Phenergan) about ten minutes before you take DHE. If you get stomach upset or heartburn but no nausea, try an antacid like Rolaids or Tums.

Flushed feeling or heat in the head, or leg cramps or aching in the legs, are common sensations. The nasal spray can cause nasal congestion.

Muscle tension, mild headache, and tightness in the chest or throat may occur briefly. Numbness or burning at the injection site may be prevented by icing the area before the injection. Diarrhea lasting about a day may occur, especially with intravenous administration.

HEADACHE HELP TIP: WATCH THAT GRAPEFRUIT JUICE

Grapefruit juice may make certain drugs stay in your system longer than they should. By inhibiting an enzyme that helps metabolize some drugs (sedatives, antianxiety agents, calcium blockers, certain statins [prescribed for high cholesterol], and antidepressants), grapefruit juice can aggravate side effects and render the drugs more potent and dangerous. Grapefruit juice should also be avoided with certain antibiotics (erythromycin, azithromycin, and clarithromycin). These lists are by no means complete.

ANTINAUSEA MEDICATION

Nausea may occur not only as a side effect of a migraine, but as a side effect of medication as well. If you are susceptible to nausea, you may want to keep some antinausea medication on hand. Most of these drugs are sedating, which many migraine sufferers find helpful. The pills are less effective than the suppositories, which are less effective than injections you can give yourself. If you experience severe nausea, keep both pills and suppositories on hand.

QUICK REFERENCE GUIDE: ANTINAUSEA MEDICATIONS

1. **OTC ANTACIDS, VITAMIN B$_6$, OR EMETROL**
    Gentle medications you can buy without a doctor's prescription.
2. **PROMETHAZINE (PHENERGAN)**
    Mild and effective yet very sedating.
3. **PROCHLORPERAZINE (COMPAZINE)**
    Very effective, but anxiety, sedation, and/or agitation are common.
4. **METOCLOPRAMIDE (REGLAN)**
    Mild, but well tolerated; mild fatigue or anxiety common.
5. **TRIMETHOBENZAMIDE (TIGAN AND OTHERS)**
    Less effective than others but well tolerated and useful in children. Lozenges can be made by some pharmacies.
6. **CHLORPROMAZINE (THORAZINE)**
    Extremely effective, but lasting sedation is common. Used when other antinausea drugs have failed.
7. **ONDANSETRON (ZOFRAN)**
    Nonsedating, few side effects, but expensive.

---

1. OVER-THE-COUNTER ANTACIDS, VITAMIN B$_6$, OR EMETROL

These preparations are available without a doctor's prescription and include antacids such as Tums, Rolaids, or Mylanta. They can sometimes help settle your stomach during a migraine.

Vitamin B_6 occasionally helps, but limit yourself to one tablet a day. Sometimes, ginger is useful for combating nausea.

Emetrol, an over-the-counter antinausea medication, may help alleviate migraine nausea. It is a phosphorated carbohydrate solution (also called Calm-X, Naus-a-way, and Nausea-tol). One or two tablets every three or four hours, as needed, are usually recommended.

2. PROMETHAZINE (PHENERGAN)

Though mild and effective, promethazine can have a strong sedative effect and will often make you fall asleep; this effect, however, may be just what you want. Safe for children, the medication may cause sudden, involuntary jerking movements (extrapyramidal side effects), but they are temporary and rare and shouldn't cause concern. Promethazine is available as a pill or a suppository, and some pharmacists will make them into oral lozenges.

TYPICAL DOSE: 25 to 50 mg by mouth or in a suppository, every three to four hours, as needed.

SIDE EFFECTS: In addition to fatigue, promethazine occasionally makes you feel dizzy or lowers your blood pressure.

3. PROCHLORPERAZINE (COMPAZINE)

Compazine is a very effective antinausea medication but produces side effects — somewhat more frequently than the other antinausea medications.

In addition to being available in long-acting pill form and suppositories, Compazine can be taken intravenously and sometimes helps to relieve pain.

TYPICAL DOSE: 10 to 25 mg by mouth, 5 or 25 mg in suppositories, or 5 to 10 mg by injection, every three to four hours, but no more than 60 mg a day.

SIDE EFFECTS: Involuntary movements, anxiety and agitation, fatigue.

4. Metoclopramide (Reglan)

Because Reglan is well tolerated, with only mild side effects, it is commonly used before IV DHE, which may be given in an emergency room for quick relief of severe pain. Adding Reglan to aspirin or an NSAID can enhance the effect, because Reglan boosts the absorption of NSAIDs and aspirin.

TYPICAL DOSE: 5 to 10 mg every four hours, as needed, but no more than 30 mg a day.

SIDE EFFECTS: Mild fatigue or anxiety and restlessness, occasional involuntary jerking.

5. Trimethobenzamide (Tigan, Arrestin, Benzacot, Bio-Gan, Stemetic, Tebamide, Tegamide, Ticon, Tigect-20, Triban, Tribenzagan)

Tigan is somewhat less effective than the other antiemetics (antinausea medications) but may be prescribed for children and has few and minimal side effects.

Tigan is available in pills and suppositories, and some pharmacists will make oral lozenges.

TYPICAL DOSE: 250 mg by mouth or as a suppository or injection, every three hours, as needed.

SIDE EFFECTS: Fatigue, occasional involuntary jerking, dizziness, blurred vision, and low blood pressure.

6. Chlorpromazine (Thorazine, Promapar, Sonazine)

Although this medication is the most effective one for relieving nausea, it has more side effects than other antiemetics and is usually reserved for when they fail. The medication also helps with pain, however, and the suppositories can often prevent a trip to the emergency room by sedating you, inducing sleep, and thereby stopping the nausea.

TYPICAL DOSE: 25 to 50 mg by mouth or in a suppository, every three hours, as needed.

SIDE EFFECTS: Long-lasting sedation. May also cause dizziness and, occasionally, involuntary jerking and slurred speech.

7. ONDANSETRON (ZOFRAN, ZOFRAN ODT)

This nonsedating antinausea medication, used primarily for cancer patients receiving chemotherapy, is highly effective, with remarkably few side effects. It rarely causes the sedation that the other antinausea medications bring on. However, it is expensive. Zofran ODT dissolves on the tongue.

TYPICAL DOSE: One tablet (4 or 8 mg) every six to eight hours, as needed.

SIDE EFFECTS: Though rare, nervousness, diarrhea, or constipation may occur.

CASE STUDIES

Here are two sample case studies to show you how a doctor might manage occasional migraines with abortive medications. Although many cases are simple, we have chosen two complex ones to take you through the rational trial-and-error process that a headache doctor might use.

DANIEL

INITIAL VISIT: Daniel, a hard-driving executive, is forty-three years old and has had migraines for twelve years. His father and grandfather also had migraines. He is a perfectionist in his work and suffers from very cold hands and feet. He has a history of motion sickness as a child, and his eyes are very sensitive to light.

Daniel reports that none of the over-the-counter medications have helped his migraines, which are so severe that they keep him from functioning. Because he suffers from only two a month, Daniel's doctor does not place him on daily preventive medication. However, because his migraines are severe, last two days, and are accompanied by nausea and vomiting, they discuss daily preventive medication as a possibility for the future. (Patients who find such medication worthwhile usually have four to five migraines a month or chronic daily tension headaches.) Daniel does not have significant risk factors for heart problems.

The doctor first briefs Daniel on the importance of watching for

headache triggers and using relaxation methods. Then he prescribes Compazine suppositories for the nausea and Imitrex Nasal
Spray for the headache. As an alternative, if Imitrex is not effective, the doctor also gives Daniel Esgic (butalbital, caffeine, and
acetaminophen) as a painkiller. (He warns Daniel that the generic
painkillers, particularly the butalbital-type medications, may not
work as well as the brand names.)

WEEK 1: Daniel calls to say that the Imitrex helped relieve his
headache, but only approximately 50 percent. The Compazine did
stop the nausea, but it made him feel nervous and agitated. The
doctor then prescribes Imitrex injections and teaches Daniel how
to use these. The doctor also changes Daniel's nausea medication
to Phenergan, which generally does not cause the nervousness associated with Compazine. However, Phenergan can cause excessive tiredness.

WEEK 5: Daniel calls to say the Imitrex injections relieve the
headache by about 90 percent, but he has tightness in the muscles
of his jaw and neck and wishes to try something else. The Esgic
has not helped. The doctor prescribes Maxalt MLT tablets for
Daniel to put on his tongue during a migraine.

WEEK 8: Daniel comes in to the doctor's office and reports
that Maxalt MLT is moderately effective, cutting his pain by
about half, but says that he would prefer going back to the Imitrex
Nasal Spray. The Phenergan is useful for the severe nausea. Daniel
and the doctor decide to use Imitrex Nasal Spray for most of the
headaches, but injections for extremely severe migraines with severe nausea. The doctor explains that it's common to have two,
three, or even more abortive medications on hand. This gives patients options to choose from for particular headaches at particular times.

THE FUTURE: If Daniel later reports that he is losing control
of his headaches, other possibilities include ergotamines (particularly suppositories), DHE injections or Migranal Nasal Spray,
Toradol injections (Toradol is the only anti-inflammatory available as an injection), or as an absolute last resort, a strong painkiller such as Stadol Nasal Spray.

DOROTHY

INITIAL VISIT: Dorothy is a thirty-nine-year-old lawyer who gets severe migraines about twice a month; they last for two days each. She gets no relief from various over-the-counter medications and relaxation-biofeedback methods. With previous physicians, she tried naproxen (Anaprox) and Norgesic Forte, neither of which were particularly helpful. The migraines are triggered occasionally by weather changes or stress, but 80 percent of the time the headaches do not have any identifiable trigger (as is the case for most people). Visits to a chiropractor, massage therapist, and acupuncturist have failed to provide any relief. Dorothy is very reluctant to use a daily preventive medication. She simply wishes to treat the headaches once they occur with an abortive medication.

Dorothy's doctor first instructs her on basic nonmedication techniques such as lying down in a dark room and applying ice packs to her head. He prescribes Midrin and Fiorinal and tells Dorothy to try them separately and together.

WEEK 3: Dorothy reports that the Midrin and Fiorinal help about 25 percent, but leave her fatigued and washed out. Dorothy's doctor prescribes Zomig as an abortive.

WEEK 6: Dorothy calls to say that the Zomig does help but makes her very nauseated. The doctor switches the medication to Imitrex Nasal Spray. He also discusses the possibility of Imitrex injections, but Dorothy wishes to wait on this approach.

The doctor also prescribes dexamethasone (Decadron), a cortisone preparation that helps shorten severe prolonged migraines. In some patients, cortisone may be the only effective abortive medication. Dorothy finds that the Imitrex Nasal Spray helps about 50 percent but leaves a slightly bad taste in her mouth. She is willing to accept this because of the headache relief. The dexamethasone irritates her stomach but shortens the headache to one day only.

WEEK 24: Dorothy says that the Imitrex Nasal Spray is no longer effective, and the headaches have become extremely severe in intensity. The doctor prescribes Stadol Nasal Spray, which does relieve some of the pain but leaves Dorothy unable to function. She does not like how she feels when she takes it. The dexamethasone continues to provide some relief and shorten the length of the headache. Dorothy's doctor now prescribes Imitrex injections and teaches Dorothy how to use them.

WEEK 26:   Dorothy calls to say that the Imitrex was helpful but made her chest feel heavy. This side effect was mild and only lasted fifteen minutes, and Dorothy does not have risk factors for heart attack. Dorothy has lost her medical insurance and says she'd like to try an inexpensive medication now. The doctor prescribes ergotamine with caffeine in tablet form.

WEEK 29:   The ergotamine tablets provide relief, but Dorothy is extremely anxious and nauseated from them. The doctor now replaces the tablets with ergotamine and caffeine PB suppositories (one-third suppository to be used every four to six hours as needed) because these generally produce much less nausea and are more effective than the tablets. The PB portion offsets the anxiety that can occur with ergotamine and caffeine.

WEEK 32:   The suppositories are somewhat effective, but the nausea remains a problem. Dorothy wishes to go back to the Imitrex injections. The Decadron has remained effective at diminishing the length of time of the headache. Dorothy continues on Imitrex injections and Decadron as needed.

THE FUTURE: If Dorothy needs to try another abortive medication, other painkillers such as hydrocodone, Fiorinal with codeine, or meperidine are possibilities; she may also use another form of triptan such as Maxalt MLT. Because she only gets two migraines a month, she does not necessarily need preventive medication, although some patients with two severe, prolonged migraines per month find preventives worthwhile. Using preventives is a possibility for Dorothy. Other possibilities would include Migranal Nasal Spray, which is DHE, or DHE injections that she could administer at home. Toradol injections, which are the only anti-inflammatories available as an injection, would be another possible remedy.

6

· · · · · · · ·

PREVENTING MIGRAINES

IT'S ONE THING to have mastered the techniques for bailing yourself out of a migraine if one starts, but an important long-term goal is learning how to prevent your migraines *before* they start. One way to achieve this goal is to identify which triggers most affect you. Another is to take a preventive medication if you get migraines frequently.

To use this chapter most efficiently, track your migraines with the Headache Calendar in Chapter 2. Every time a headache comes on, try to identify which factor on the list might have played a role in triggering it. Highlight a handful of potential triggers and do all you can to eliminate them from your life. See if the headaches improve. Reintroduce the potential triggers one at a time. Later in this chapter, we will discuss preventive medications to use when the nondrug strategies don't work well enough.

RECOGNIZING COMMON TRIGGERS

Many factors have been identified as possible migraine triggers, but most people are sensitive to only a few. Unfortunately, however, what triggers a headache today won't necessarily be what brings one on next week. Also, the different elements to which you are sensitive can gang up and give you a terrible headache even when they might not have affected you individually. A sudden weather change compounded by job stress, for example, may be enough to take you over the edge. Not everyone can isolate the primary headache culprits, but others, through experience, do notice specific patterns. The more observant you are in identifying your patterns, the better off you'll be. Be mindful of these potential triggers:

COMMON MIGRAINE TRIGGERS

- Overwhelming "daily hassles"
- Stress, worry, depression, anxiety, and anger
- Some foods
- Weather and seasonal changes, such as high humidity or high heat
- Smoke, perfume, gasoline, paint, organic solvents, and other strong odors
- Hunger
- Fatigue or lack of sleep
- Hormonal factors, such as menstruation, birth control pills, pregnancy, menopause, estrogens
- Oversleeping and excessive sleep
- Exertion, exercise, or sex
- Bright lights, such as glaring artificial lights or bright sunlight
- Head trauma
- Altitude
- Motion, experienced during long car rides or amusement park rides, for example

"DAILY HASSLES," STRESS, WORRY, DEPRESSION, ANXIETY, AND ANGER

"Bad stress" or negative emotions aren't the only contributors to headaches. Too many daily problems, particularly after a bad day or a poor night's sleep, can exacerbate them as well. Although emotions do not *cause* migraines, which are an inherited, physical illness, certain emotions can *trigger* migraines. Any problem — trouble at work, illness in the family, financial woes, bickering with a loved one — that causes stress may bring on a headache.

That's not to say that the headache is psychological; rather, the stress causes complex biochemical changes in the body that can disrupt your equilibrium, and cause your neck, shoulders, and head muscles to tighten up, thereby triggering your susceptible headache mechanism.

For some people, stress itself triggers a migraine. In others, however, the letdown period that occurs after a stressful event or period precipitates a headache. Monday-to-Friday workers, for example, often suffer from weekend headaches. Migraine-free through the workweek, they may suffer from a letdown headache as soon as the weekend begins and the stressful week is over. Weekend headaches, as we've discussed, may also be due to caffeine withdrawal.

Depression may trigger migraines, but again, it does not cause them. As you may have experienced, suffering from severe, recurring head pain can be depressing. Recent studies have suggested that if you get migraines, you may also be at greater risk for depression and anxiety, probably because all these conditions are related to the neurotransmitter serotonin. As a result, if you do get depressed or emotionally stressed, chances are your headaches will continue until these problems are resolved.

A most effective way to resolve troubling emotions is with psychotherapy, which can teach you how to deal better with problems and to use relaxation methods to help mitigate the potentially damaging effects of stress. By helping you learn how to resolve conflicts with other people, modify perfectionist behavior, and deal with anger and other repressed emotions, you may actually find that your migraines diminish in intensity and frequency.

So don't be offended if your doctor suggests psychotherapy; such a recommendation does not imply that the pain is all in your head, but is intended to suggest the potential vast benefits of psychotherapy and stress management. Too few people put in the time, effort, and money necessary to try just a few sessions with a psychotherapist to learn specific coping and relaxation skills, which can be a powerful ally in their fight against headaches. (These strategies and techniques are discussed in detail in Chapter 2.) Learning to accept your headache situation and accept that there is no cure (though there *is* effective treatment) helps ease anxiety about headaches, which in turn can be therapeutic. You are not causing your headaches, nor should you be blamed for them.

SOME FOODS

More than 25 percent of migraine sufferers can identify foods that trigger an attack. Note that if a specific food provokes a headache in you, this reaction is probably not an allergic one, contrary to the views of many people, but rather a sensitivity to specific chemicals in these foods: amines (in aged cheese, pickled herring, and bananas); phenylethylamine (in chocolate); monosodium glutamate, or MSG (in Chinese food); and nitrites (in luncheon meats, bacon, and hot dogs). The chemical may trigger a migraine because of its effect on the brain or blood vessels, which is very different from an allergic reaction.

Although food-triggered headaches often start soon after eating, several hours may go by before onset. Also, you may be sensitive to the offending food only sometimes. Women, for example, may be particularly sensitive around their menstrual periods. And remember, triggers are "additive"; one food may not cause a headache, but two offending foods may.

Study the food list that follows, and if you have a hunch about certain foods to avoid, omit them from your diet for at least several weeks. If you have no idea where to start, avoid them all or choose a few. Gradually add back one food at a time, noting which ones may be headache culprits. Don't become frustrated or disappointed if you watch the foods carefully but still get headaches. Food is but one of many influencing factors and, compared to stress and biochemical imbalances, a relatively minor one.

COMMON MIGRAINE FOOD TRIGGERS

- Alcohol (less than the amount consumed to cause a hangover), most commonly red wine, as well as brandy, whiskey, champagne, white wine, beer, and other drinks
- Chocolate and chocolate milk, cocoa
- Cheese, ripened, such as Cheddar, blue, brick, Colby, Roquefort, Brie, Gruyère, mozzarella, Parmesan, Boursault, and Romano; and processed, though American cheese, along with cottage cheese and cream cheese, is much less likely to trigger a headache than the aged cheeses
- Citrus fruit, including grapefruit and orange
- Pineapple
- Caffeine in coffee, soda, cocoa, and other drinks. (Usually caffeine helps headaches; too much caffeine, though, can cause increased, rebound headaches. Heavy caffeine users need to reduce their intake gradually. Some migraine sufferers are extremely sensitive to small amounts of caffeine. See Chapter 2 for amounts of caffeine in common foods and drinks.)
- Monosodium glutamate (MSG) may also be labeled "autolyzed yeast extract," "hydrolyzed vegetable protein," or "natural flavoring." Possible sources of MSG include Chinese restaurant food; broth or stock; canned or instant soup; whey protein; soy extract; malt extract; caseinate; barley extract; textured soy protein; chicken, pork, or beef flavoring; processed meat; smoke flavor; spices and seasonings, including seasoned salt; carrageenan; meat tenderizer; TV dinners; instant gravy; and some potato chips and dry-roasted nuts.
- Hot dog, pepperoni, bologna, salami, sausage, canned or aged meat, cured meat (bacon, ham), or marinated meat
- Fresh, hot homemade yeast bread (once cool it is OK)
- Buttermilk
- Yeast extract
- Acidophilus milk

- Pizza, freshly baked and still hot (less likely to trigger headache if cooled and reheated)
- Aspartame, such as NutraSweet, a popular artificial sweetener

---

HEADACHE HELP TIP: WHAT TO DRINK IF YOU MUST DRINK

If you really want to drink, your best bet is to have no more than two normal-size drinks and choose one of the following, which are less likely to trigger a migraine: a Sauternes or Riesling wine; Seagram's VO whiskey or Cutty Sark scotch. Of all alcohol, vodka is the least likely to set off a headache.

LESS COMMON MIGRAINE FOOD TRIGGERS

- Onions
- Beans, such as lima, navy, fava, lentil, garbanzo, pinto, and Italian
- Snow peas
- Sauerkraut
- Pickles and pickled food
- Marinades
- Chili peppers
- Licorice or carob candy
- Figs, raisins, avocados, bananas, passion fruit, papayas
- Fried food
- Peanut, peanut butter
- Popcorn
- Nuts or seeds, all types
- Soy sauce
- Sugar in excess
- Salt in excess
- Seafood
- Sour cream or yogurt
- Pork and chicken liver

WEATHER AND SEASONAL CHANGES

Spring tends to be the worst season for migraine sufferers, then fall. The hot humid days of summer may also be bad. You may be sensitive to weather changes, regardless of the season, because such changes can alter the body's chemical balance. Weather tends to affect the severity, not the frequency, of migraines. Although research on weather and headache produces conflicting results, more often than not weather emerges as a major trigger. However, most weather triggers for migraines can't be pinpointed to any single identifiable cause.

SMOKE, PERFUME, GASOLINE, PAINT, ORGANIC SOLVENTS

Certain people are particularly sensitive to these substances. Sensitivity to cigarette smoke may develop anytime, even in people who used to be smokers. Many people cannot stand to be exposed to even small amounts of perfumes or gasoline. Magazines that contain perfume are often a hazard for the migraine-prone (subscription magazines may be ordered without them); paint smells are also common triggers for migraines.

HUNGER

Most people who get migraines recognize that if they miss meals they are more likely to get a headache. If this is true for you, be sure to eat regularly, at least three times a day. Anticipate periods when there may not be food available (when traveling, for example) and be sure to bring a snack.

FATIGUE OR LACK OF SLEEP

Children who get migraines are especially sensitive to lack of sleep. Other migraine sufferers who are awakened early in the morning, particularly by a bright light (sun shining through an uncovered window), often experience a migraine. People who must change time shifts for their jobs often experience migraines during the adjustment period. Whenever possible, be consistent with your sleep habits.

HORMONAL FACTORS

Menstruation, especially, but also birth control pills, pregnancy, menopause, and estrogen supplements often play a crucial role in triggering migraines in women. Menstrual migraines often are the most severe and tend to be the most difficult to treat. Headaches are sometimes better during pregnancy, at least in the last two trimesters. (See Chapter 7 for detailed information on the relationship between hormones and migraines in women.)

OVERSLEEPING AND EXCESSIVE SLEEP

Although most children and adolescents are unaffected by oversleeping, too much sleep in adults can lead to a migraine attack. Be careful about regulating your sleep, especially on weekends. Naps can also be a problem. Even just a half hour of extra sleep on a Sunday morning, after a stressful week, may be enough to trigger a migraine.

EXERTION, EXERCISE, OR SEX

For some people, certain types of exertion, including sex, consistently trigger a migraine. Anti-inflammatories taken before exercising or having sex often prevent the headache. (See Chapter 13 for more on exertion and sex headaches.)

BRIGHT LIGHTS

If you get migraines, chances are you are sensitive to bright fluorescent light and sunlight, even when you don't have a headache. Wearing sunglasses can help; be sure to keep a spare pair in the car because windshield glare is a common trigger. Many migraine sufferers are also bothered by oncoming headlights at night. Camera flashes, fluorescent lights in grocery stores, and too much time in front of a computer screen are also triggers. Anti-glare screens (and taking frequent breaks) may ease computer-related headaches.

HEAD TRAUMA

A blow to the head can cause migraines whether or not you have a history of migraine headaches. Rear-end whiplash accidents are common triggers, and the related migraines may persist for months or years. (See Chapter 13 for more on post-traumatic headaches.)

ALTITUDE

Some people get migraines at high altitudes. One reason may be that there is less oxygen high up, and the blood vessels in the body try to compensate by dilating, a cause of headache in some people. Exercise may help by getting more oxygen into the blood. Vitamin C might also help ward off the effects of high altitudes. Sometimes special medications, such as a water pill called Diamox or steroids, can help too.

MOTION

Sometimes travel by car, plane, train, or boat can trigger a migraine for reasons that researchers can't explain. Some children who get motion sickness develop migraines several years later. Preventing motion sickness by riding in the front seat and making frequent road stops may help ward off a potential migraine.

PREVENTING MIGRAINES WITH MEDICATIONS

If you suffer from frequent headaches and the strategies discussed so far are not adequate to relieve them, your doctor may recommend preventive medications, though the ultimate decision to try them will be yours. Think about the fact, however, that you will probably end up taking less medication for migraine prevention than if you simply chase after frequent headaches with pain relievers.

Consider preventive medication if:

1. You get moderate to severe migraines more than three times a month.
2. The medications to relieve the migraines fail to provide adequate relief.
3. Your quality of life is sufficiently compromised by migraine severity or frequency.
4. You are willing to take medication daily, accept that possible side effects may occur, and change medications if necessary.
5. You have daily, or near-daily, headaches in addition to migraines.
6. You have other conditions that could be helped with a daily preventive medication. For instance, if you are anxious or depressed, antidepressants could help prevent headaches and the anxiety and depression; high blood pressure could be lowered by beta- or calcium blockers and help prevent headaches. If you have arthritis, anti-inflammatories could help ease it and your headaches.

Although these medications won't usually completely eliminate migraines, they usually significantly reduce the overall impact that migraines have on your life. A trial course of about four weeks is necessary before you can assess a medication's usefulness.

Choosing a preventive medication will depend on factors such as whether you also get chronic tension headaches, your age, sensitivity to side effects, sleeping patterns, stomach sensitivity, blood pressure, pulse, and other medical concerns.

Starting on preventive medication will take some patience and perseverance. Here are some general guidelines:

UNDERSTAND THE GOAL

Although it would be great if you could eliminate 90 to 100 percent of your migraines, that would probably require too much medication with too many side effects. Your goal for reducing migraine frequency, therefore, must be modified to a realistic 50 to 90 percent improvement; your goal for reducing the intensity or severity of your migraines should be a realistic 70 percent improvement.

BE WILLING TO CHANGE

Be open to changing medications if one doesn't work or causes too many side effects. And remember that what worked for someone else won't necessarily work for you.

BE TOLERANT

Try to be willing to endure mildly annoying side effects in order to achieve positive results with the headaches.

BE PATIENT

Many of the medications need several weeks to become fully effective, and doses may need to be adjusted. Call your doctor if you have problems or concerns, but try to stick with each medication for the desired length of time.

BE WELL INFORMED

Most of these medications are used for other health conditions besides headache. Learn what they are and why you are using the drug for headache. Be aware of possible side effects so you are not frightened or confused if they occur. Consult the *Physicians' Desk Reference* to learn about risks associated with any medication.

FIRST-LINE MEDICATIONS FOR PREVENTING MIGRAINES

QUICK REFERENCE GUIDE: FIRST-LINE MEDICATIONS FOR PREVENTING MIGRAINES

1. **DEPAKOTE**
   Very effective and safe, but fatigue and weight gain may occur.
2. **ANTIDEPRESSANTS (ELAVIL, ZOLOFT, PAXIL, SINEQUAN, VIVACTIL, NORPRAMIN, AND SO ON)**
   Effective, inexpensive, and also useful for daily headaches

---

and insomnia. Some of these drugs cause sedation, weight gain, dry mouth, and constipation. (See Table, page 111.)

3. **BETA-BLOCKERS (INDERAL, LOPRESSOR, CORGARD, TENORMIN)**

Effective, though sedation, diarrhea, lower gastrointestinal (GI) upset, and weight gain are common. Very useful in combination with amitriptyline.

4. **NSAIDs (NAPROSYN, NAPRELAN, ALEVE, ANAPROX, ANSAID, ORUDISKT, ORUVAIL, VOLTAREN, CATAFLAM, CELEBREX, VIOXX)**

Particularly useful for menstrual migraine. Nonsedating, but frequent GI upset (except for Celebrex and Vioxx).

5. **CALCIUM BLOCKERS (ISOPTIN, CALAN, VERELAN)**

Less effective, but fewer side effects, except for constipation; usually nonsedating and don't cause weight gain.

---

1. DEPAKOTE

Depakote is now one of the primary headache preventive medications because it's very effective for migraine and daily headaches. Depakote is also prescribed for certain types of seizures, and as a "mood stabilizer" for anxiety and depression in people with bipolar illness (manic-depression). Antidepressants, calcium blockers, or beta-blockers may be taken in conjunction with Depakote. As with most medications, smaller doses of Depakote are prescribed for headaches than for other conditions, such as seizures.

TYPICAL DOSE: 250 mg a day to start, with food, increased over days to an average dose of 500 mg once or twice a day (sometimes up to 1,500 or 2,000 mg a day). It takes at least four or five weeks to know if Depakote will work. Blood tests (to check your liver) will occasionally be necessary. However, Depakote has generally been a very safe medication, particularly in low doses.

SIDE EFFECTS: Fatigue and weight gain, although no side effects may occur. Nausea, stomach upset, and sedation sometimes also occur. With higher doses, hair loss or a tremor in the hand may occur. These tend to be related to the dose and may subside if the dose is lowered. Do not use Depakote if you might be pregnant.

2. ANTIDEPRESSANTS

Although these medications are commonly used at high doses to combat depression, that's not why they are recommended here. Some of these drugs, such as amitriptyline and other similar so-called tricyclic antidepressants, are useful because they tend to increase the concentration of serotonin in the brain. Newer antidepressants, which are not tricyclics, like Prozac, Zoloft, and Paxil, also influence serotonin.

Prozac, Zoloft, Paxil, and the other newer antidepressants are somewhat less effective for pain than the older ones, such as amitriptyline. However, these newer medications have considerably fewer side effects and are more effective for anxiety and depression in low doses than the older drugs. They are all helpful for chronic daily headache as well. All of these antidepressants are useful for panic disorder. In addition, they are used in people with bipolar illness (manic-depression), usually in conjunction with a "mood stabilizer," such as Depakote or lithium.

Prozac, Zoloft, and Paxil have been widely used for at least ten years now, and the fears for long-term side effects are diminishing. While no long-term side effects have been identified, it may take decades before we can definitely say that they are completely safe for the long term. However, tens of millions of people have been on these medications for long periods of time.

Note: Many of these medications can influence heart rate, increasing the risk of a rapid heartbeat. For that reason, they are prescribed with caution for the elderly and are sometimes used with a beta-blocker (the next group of drugs we'll discuss) to lower the pulse rate.

- ### AMITRIPTYLINE (ELAVIL)

This is the most commonly prescribed antidepressant because it is effective, inexpensive, and can help you sleep. It is particularly useful if you get both daily tension headaches and migraines.

TYPICAL DOSE: It is important to begin with only 10 mg, which may be all many people can tolerate, taken at night, working up to 25 or 50 mg (doses far below those used to treat depression) in several weeks. The dose can be pushed up to 150 or 200 mg if needed. Some people do well with as little as 5 mg (half a tablet).

SIDE EFFECTS: Sedation (which decreases over time), weight gain, a dry mouth (which can be countered with Oral Balance Gel or Biotene toothpaste), constipation, dizziness. Occasional anxiety or nervousness, which will usually decrease in time. Less common side effects are depression, blurred vision, memory difficulties, and insomnia (although usually amitriptyline induces sleepiness).

- **FLUOXETINE (PROZAC)**

A very well-tolerated antidepressant that is less effective for pain but has far fewer side effects than amitriptyline and the other older antidepressants.

TYPICAL DOSE: Doctors begin with a low dose of these medications and watch for any anxiety or nervousness that may occur. After several days or a week, however, these reactions usually stop. These medications are excellent in treating anxiety and nervousness, but in the beginning they may actually exacerbate them. With Prozac, doctors usually begin with half a 10-mg tablet in the morning, and then, if necessary, increase the dose to 20 mg or higher over days to weeks. The key is to begin with low doses. Prozac is available in 10-mg, 20-mg, and 40-mg capsules and 10-mg tablets; liquid Prozac is also available.

SIDE EFFECTS: Initial anxiety or nervousness is relatively common. Insomnia, a feeling of spaciness, and fatigue may occur. Occasionally, people experience sweating, weight loss or weight gain, or tremors. If you are extremely agitated or up all night with these medications, it is best to stop them and call your physician.

Sexual side effects (decreased ability or decreased sex drive) are relatively common with many antidepressants. Prozac, Zoloft, and Paxil cause these sexual side effects in many people. In fact, they are one of the main reasons why people discontinue taking them. Minimizing the dose is crucial for minimizing the side effects. The antidepressant Wellbutrin (see section below on Miscellaneous Antidepressants) tends to cause fewer sexual side effects.

- **SERTRALINE (ZOLOFT)**

Similar to Prozac, Zoloft is extremely well tolerated and very useful for anxiety, depression, and chronic daily headaches. However, these newer antidepressants are less effective for pain and headaches than amitriptyline and the other older (tricyclic) antidepressants. Some people tolerate Prozac but do poorly on Zoloft, and vice versa. You may want to try several of these antidepressants, therefore, before you give up on them.

TYPICAL DOSE: One or half a 25-mg tablet to start, increasing over four to six days to 50 mg. The usual dose for headaches is low, 25 mg to 75 mg per day. For depression, 75 mg to 150 mg (or more) is often prescribed. Zoloft is available in conveniently scored tablets of 25-mg, 50-mg, and 100-mg doses, and may be taken once per day. With most of these medications, all of the doses are the same price, so using a higher strength tablet and cutting it in half is usually less expensive.

SIDE EFFECTS: Similar to Prozac — generally milder than the older (tricyclic) antidepressants.

- **PAROXETINE (PAXIL)**

Very similar to Prozac and Zoloft, Paxil is also available in very convenient scored tablets of 10-mg, 20-mg, 30-mg, and 40-mg doses. Paxil is very well tolerated, but if you are on more than 10 mg per day and suddenly stop the medication, you may experience mild withdrawal symptoms for two or three days. These symptoms are flulike feelings, with tiredness.

As with the others antidepressants, Paxil is very useful in some patients for chronic daily headache, and of course, for anxiety or depression.

TYPICAL DOSE: One or half a 10-mg tablet, for four to six days, increasing slowly to 20 mg per day. The usual dose for headaches is low, 10 mg to 30 mg per day. The usual depression dose is 30 mg or 40 mg (or more) daily. It is crucial to begin with low doses.

SIDE EFFECTS: Similar to Prozac.

- **DOXEPIN (SINEQUAN)**

Very similar to amitriptyline, doxepin is extremely helpful for migraines and tension headaches, as well as anxiety.

TYPICAL DOSE: Usually begins with only 10 mg, to be taken at night, which is all that many people can tolerate; if tolerated, the dose may be slowly increased to 50 or 75 mg and up to 150 mg or more, but if 150 mg is not effective, the medication should probably be changed. A typical dose is 50 mg.

SIDE EFFECTS: Sedation, weight gain, a dry mouth, dizziness, and constipation. (See side effects for amitriptyline for more detail.)

- **NORTRIPTYLINE (PAMELOR, AVENTYL)**

When amitriptyline has been effective, but its side effects are too severe, doctors sometimes recommend nortriptyline because it causes less sedation; however, it is less effective and more expensive than amitriptyline. Nortriptyline is safer for the elderly than amitriptyline and the other older antidepressants because it has a relatively low risk of cardiac side effects. The new antidepressants, such as Prozac, however, may be even safer. Nortriptyline is also useful for children and adolescents.

TYPICAL DOSE: 10 mg to start, slowly increasing to 25 mg, sometimes to 100 mg, taken at night. Only available as capsules.

SIDE EFFECTS: Similar to amitriptyline but less severe, including sedation (which decreases over time), weight gain, a dry mouth, constipation, or dizziness. Occasional anxiety or nervousness, but these side effects will quickly decrease. Less common side effects are depression, blurred vision, memory difficulties, and insomnia.

- **PROTRIPTYLINE (VIVACTIL)**

Protriptyline is often used when tension headaches are also a problem, or when nortriptyline's side effects, such as sedation and weight gain, are too severe. It is not sedating and does not cause weight gain.

TYPICAL DOSE: 2.5 mg to start each morning, increasing to 5 or 10 mg (sometimes even 30 or 50 mg, the typical doses prescribed for depression).

SIDE EFFECTS: Nervousness. A dry mouth, constipation, and dizziness may occur. Insomnia (countered by taking it in the morning) occurs often, blurred vision and stomach upset less often.

- **DESIPRAMINE (NORPRAMIN)**

  Milder than other antidepressants, desipramine is useful if you are very sensitive to drug side effects. This medication is much more helpful, however, for chronic daily headaches than for migraines (see Chapter 9).

- **TRIMIPRAMINE (SURMONTIL)**

  Trimipramine is a good choice when amitriptyline no longer works or if its side effects are too severe. Though well tolerated compared to the other antidepressants, it is sedating. It is usually much more helpful for daily headaches than for migraines (see Chapter 9).

There are other antidepressants, known as MAO inhibitor antidepressants, such as phenelzine (Nardil), which are extremely effective, but their side effects, especially insomnia and weight gain, are severe compared with other antidepressants. Also, if you take an MAO inhibitor antidepressant, you will have to observe a very strict diet for safety reasons.

- **MISCELLANEOUS ANTIDEPRESSANTS (WELLBUTRIN, REMERON, EFFEXOR, SERZONE)**

  Various other antidepressants are sometimes prescribed to prevent daily headache, migraine, or the anxiety and depression that often accompany chronic headaches.

  Wellbutrin (bupropion) is a well-tolerated older antidepressant that rarely causes the sedation, weight gain, and sexual dysfunction often seen with other antidepressants. The usual dose is Wellbutrin SR 150 mg once or twice per day. While well tolerated and excellent for depression, Wellbutrin may not be as effective as some of the others for headache.

  Remeron (mirtazapine) is a very effective antidepressant that is also useful for insomnia. The usual dose is 15 mg or 30 mg once per day. Sedation and weight gain may become major problems, however. Remeron is one of the very effective newer antidepressants.

  Effexor (venlafaxine) is an excellent antidepressant that is occasionally useful for headache sufferers. The usual dose is

75 mg to 150 mg once per day. Nausea or dizziness may occur, but Effexor is generally well tolerated. Effexor has been a safe medication that has gained popularity for anxiety and depression in the past several years.

THE ANTIDEPRESSANTS: COMPARING SIDE EFFECTS

Drug Generic (Trade Name)	Sedation	Weight Gain	Anticholinergic Effect*
Doxepin (Sinequan)	Severe	Severe	Moderate
Amitriptyline (Elavil)	Severe	Severe	Severe
Protriptyline (Vivactil)	None	None	Severe
Fluoxetine (Prozac)	Mild	Mild	None
Sertraline (Zoloft)	Mild	Mild	None
Paroxetine (Paxil)	Mild	Mild	Mild
Nortriptyline (Pamelor, Aventyl)	Moderate	Moderate	Moderate
Desipramine (Norpramin)	Mild	Mild	Mild
Trimipramine (Surmontil)	Severe	Severe	Moderate
Citalopram (Celexa)	Mild	Mild	None
Nefazodone (Serzone)	Moderate	Mild	Mild
Bupropion (Wellbutrin)	Mild	None	None
Mirtazapine (Remeron)	Severe	Severe	Mild
Venlafaxine (Effexor)	Mild	Mild	Mild
Phenelzine (Nardil)	Mild	Very severe	Moderate

*Tendency of the medication to cause a dry mouth, constipation, difficulty urinating, heartbeat irregularities, sweating, drowsiness, dizziness, and low blood pressure upon standing up suddenly. With the exception of a dry mouth and constipation, other symptoms are relatively rare.

Serzone (nefazodone) is an effective newer antidepressant useful for insomnia as well. It is relatively mild, with typical antidepressant doses ranging from 200 mg to 450 mg. For headache sufferers, doctors typically recommend lower doses, such as 100 mg to 200 mg, at night. Serzone is relatively well tolerated, though sedation and weight gain may occur; occasionally helps headaches as well as anxiety or depression.

3. BETA-BLOCKERS

Beta-blockers, which prevent blood vessel dilation, are just as effective as amitriptyline or Depakote in preventing migraines, and often are used in combination with amitriptyline. Because they lower the pulse rate (which often gives people the sense of being slowed down), they may be prescribed with amitriptyline (or another antidepressant) to counter the antidepressant's influence in increasing the heart rate.

If you have high blood pressure, taking a beta-blocker can help both the hypertension and the migraines. Beta-blockers also tend to help counter anxiety, but they may contribute to weight gain, depression, fatigue, higher cholesterol levels, diminished interest in sex, and problems concentrating. The side effects cease once you stop taking the drug.

If one beta-blocker doesn't help, your doctor is likely to recommend another because the mechanism of action of the various beta-blockers works differently.

- **PROPRANOLOL (INDERAL)**

Inderal is by far the most widely studied and most frequently prescribed beta-blocker. It prevents blood vessel dilation and helps stabilize blood flow through a serotonin mechanism. Inderal is often prescribed with amitriptyline for optimal results.

Inderal is usually not recommended if you have asthma or congestive heart failure, and should be used with caution if you have Raynaud's syndrome, a circulatory disorder.

TYPICAL DOSE: 60 mg to start, usually maintained between 60 mg and 160 mg per day. Must taper off to discontinue (except when used in a low dose by a young person, under age thirty, for a short time). Usually, it is taken once a day, in long-acting capsule form.

SIDE EFFECTS: Because propranolol easily enters the central nervous system, side effects such as fatigue are relatively common. Diarrhea, gas, and stomach upset are also fairly common; insomnia, depression, lightheadedness, and difficulty concentrating are less common. Other possible side effects include lethargy, weight gain, less tolerance to exercising, wheezing, and shortness of breath.

- **METOPROLOL (LOPRESSOR)**

This medication occasionally works when propranolol does not. If you get chronic daily headaches as well as migraines, metoprolol may be a good choice.

TYPICAL DOSE: 25 mg to start, twice a day. This may be increased to 50 mg, twice a day. Increasing the dose gradually minimizes side effects.

SIDE EFFECTS: Same as propranolol but with fewer respiratory problems.

- **NADOLOL (CORGARD)**

Nadolol is as effective as propranolol and may work when propranolol does not.

TYPICAL DOSE: 20 mg, increased to 40 through 120 mg, per day, with most people maintaining at 80 mg and lower. The scored tablets make dosage adjustments easy.

SIDE EFFECTS: Similar to propranolol with less fatigue.

- **ATENOLOL (TENORMIN)**

Because this medication doesn't affect the lungs as much as the other beta-blockers do, this medication causes fewer breathing problems. If you have any tendency toward asthma, however, you should use atenolol only with extreme caution.

TYPICAL DOSE: 50 mg, once a day. This may be increased to 100 mg per day, if necessary.

SIDE EFFECTS: Possibly less sedation and less fatigue than with propranolol.

- **TIMOLOL (BLOCADREN)**

Timolol is also sometimes effective when the other beta-blockers have failed.

TYPICAL DOSE: To minimize side effects, this medication is usually started with 5 mg taken twice a day, then up to 20 or 30 mg twice a day if necessary.

SIDE EFFECTS: Same as propranolol, but possibly with less sedation.

4. NONSTEROIDAL ANTI-INFLAMMATORIES (NSAIDs)

The NSAIDs can be very effective for preventing migraines, but their use is limited because they tend to cause gastrointestinal distress (stomach upset or ulcers) and potentially serious liver and kidney irritation. The new class of NSAIDs, the Cox-2 inhibitors (Celebrex, Vioxx), cause much less stomach irritation and are generally deemed safe. Vioxx particularly may be a useful medication because it is indicated for acute pain, and causes fewer rashes or allergic reactions.

But for women under age forty suffering from menstrual migraines (and menstrual cramps), and for those who are under age forty and very sensitive to the side effects of the beta-blockers and antidepressants, NSAIDs may be a good choice. They also can help with arthritis or musculoskeletal problems (painful knee, back, shoulder).

If you have found NSAIDs effective as an abortive medication (to dull the pain of a migraine in progress) and your doctor recommends switching to a daily preventive medication, a lower-dose NSAID may be right for you because you know it works and that you are tolerant of its potential side effects. Remember, however, always to take these medications with food.

- **NAPROXEN (NAPRELAN, ALEVE, NAPROSYN, ANAPROX)**
  Naproxen is the most widely studied and most frequently prescribed NSAID for migraines, but it is recommended only if you are under age fifty. It can be particularly useful if you get menstrual migraines and daily headaches. Naproxen is sometimes combined with another first-line preventive medication (such as amitriptyline) to enhance effectiveness. Naprelan is an excellent, long-acting form of naproxen (available in 375 mg and 500 mg).

  TYPICAL DOSE: 500 to 550 mg once a day, sometimes twice

a day. An over-the-counter version, Aleve, is available in a lower dosage, 220 mg per tablet.

SIDE EFFECTS: The most common is stomach upset or pain. If you find that naproxen is very effective for your migraines but gives you an upset stomach, your doctor may recommend using an antacid. Usually, if side effects do occur, the NSAID will be discontinued.

Other potential side effects include skin rashes, fatigue, fluid retention (swelling of hands or feet), ringing in the ear, and tension headaches. When used chronically, the liver and kidneys need to be periodically monitored with a simple blood test.

- **FLURBIPROFEN (ANSAID)**

Well tolerated, flurbiprofen is particularly useful for menstrual headaches (see Chapter 7).

TYPICAL DOSE: 100 mg twice a day.

SIDE EFFECTS: Risk of kidney and liver irritation; must be monitored periodically with blood tests.

- **KETOPROFEN (ORUDIS, ORUVAIL, ORUDISKT)**

Ketoprofen is quite helpful in preventing migraines, and sometimes tension headaches.

TYPICAL DOSE: 75 mg to 150 mg per day. Now available as a very convenient once-a-day preparation called Oruvail (100, 150, and 200 mg).

SIDE EFFECTS: Similar to the other NSAIDs; liver and kidney blood tests should be regularly monitored.

- **COX-2 INHIBITORS (CELEBREX, VIOXX)**

These newer anti-inflammatories may prove to be useful for headaches. Safety and efficacy have not been definitively established though. Vioxx appears to be particularly useful due to fewer allergic reactions, and it's indicated for acute pain. Vioxx is available in 12.5-mg, 25-mg, and 50-mg tablets. The usual dose would be 12.5 or 25 mg once a day.

5. CALCIUM BLOCKERS

Calcium blockers are generally not as effective as antidepressants, Depakote, or beta-blockers. However, they have fewer side effects and do not usually cause the weight gain or lethargy that these other preventive medications often do. If you are an athlete or would be particularly dismayed by a beta-blocker's effect of impeding athletic performance, you may want to ask your doctor about using calcium blockers to prevent your migraines.

The primary medication prescribed in this group is verapamil, although nifedipine (Procardia) and diltiazem (Cardizem) are occasionally helpful.

- **VERAPAMIL (ISOPTIN, CALAN, VERELAN)**
  This is the most widely prescribed and most effective calcium blocker, but it may take up to six weeks to become effective. Also useful for cluster headaches, verapamil is often combined with amitriptyline or naproxen to maximize relief. If you have Raynaud's syndrome, a circulatory disorder common among migraine sufferers, then verapamil may be a particularly good choice for you as it helps counteract the problems associated with Raynaud's.

  TYPICAL DOSE: Convenient once-a-day tablet, 120 mg to start, increased to an average of 180 or 240 a day.

  SIDE EFFECTS: Relatively few other than constipation, which is very common. Occasional skin rashes, dizziness, insomnia, swelling of hands and feet, and anxiety. Fatigue is less common.

SECOND-LINE MEDICATIONS FOR PREVENTING MIGRAINES

QUICK REFERENCE GUIDE: SECOND-LINE MEDICATIONS FOR PREVENTING MIGRAINES

1. **TWO FIRST-LINE MEDICATIONS ARE USED TOGETHER.**
   Two are often more effective than one.
2. **METHYSERGIDE (SANSERT)**
   Extremely effective, but nausea, leg cramps, and dizziness are common.

---

3. GABAPENTIN (NEURONTIN)

Often useful and produces no weight gain. Often combined with a first-line preventive medication.

4. NATURAL HERBS/SUPPLEMENTS (FEVERFEW, MAGNESIUM OXIDE, VITAMIN B$_2$)

These supplements can sometimes be very useful.

1. TWO FIRST-LINE PREVENTIVE MEDICATIONS

In some cases, using two medications can be effective when each medication used individually was not. Typically, a doctor may suggest combining two preventive medications if you:

- **HAVE TRIED INDIVIDUAL MEDICATIONS, BUT THEY HAVEN'T WORKED.**

  Usually doctors prescribe one preventive medication at a time, starting with low doses and raising them slowly if needed. Most people appreciate this approach, are prepared to wait for the medications to work, and are willing to switch medications if necessary.

- **ARE EXTREMELY FRUSTRATED AND WANT FAST RESULTS.**

  When you have moderate or severe chronic daily headaches as well as bothersome migraines, you and your doctor may decide to push ahead at a faster rate with the preventive approach. Depending on how severe your headaches are and how frustrated you are with treatments, your doctor has several ways to accelerate your treatment, among them increasing your doses more quickly than usual.

- **ARE SUFFERING FROM A NEW ONSET OF SEVERE HEADACHES.**

  If you have become very upset and frustrated with head pain because your headaches seem to be worsening or becoming more frequent, the doctor may decide to push preventive medication at a faster pace.

  Typically, the doses and potential side effects of using two medications together are the same as when they are used individually. Here are some common pairings that doctors use to prevent migraines.

- **DEPAKOTE WITH ANTIDEPRESSANTS**
Depakote may be combined with antidepressants, beta-blockers, or calcium blockers. For people with bipolar illness (manic-depression), Depakote plus an antidepressant is often very effective for mood swings, anxiety, and depression. Depakote with other medications, though, may cause sedation or weight gain.

- **AMITRIPTYLINE WITH PROPRANOLOL**
When amitriptyline increases heart rate, propranolol is often added to neutralize the effect. This combination is often used when both migraines and chronic daily headaches are problems.

- **NSAID WITH ANOTHER FIRST-LINE MEDICATION**
Naproxen (or another NSAID) is often prescribed with amitriptyline (an antidepressant), propranolol (a beta-blocker), or verapamil (a calcium blocker) to serve as both preventive and abortive medications.

If you are over fifty, however, an NSAID is usually a third-line choice because of the increased risk of gastrointestinal, kidney, and liver problems.

2. METHYSERGIDE (SANSERT)

This extremely powerful preventive medication seems to help constrict swollen blood vessels and affect serotonin, but it is not commonly used because of the possible side effect of fibrosis, a "thickening" about the lungs, heart, or kidneys, which occurs in one out of seven hundred patients. With careful use and low doses, however, it can be relatively safe and effective.

Methysergide is most often prescribed for people forty-five and younger because its constricting effect on blood vessels can present a problem in older people. It is also not a good choice if you have coronary artery disease, previous blood clots (thrombophlebitis), peptic ulcers, kidney or liver problems, or any vascular disorders. If you have high blood pressure, your doctor should closely monitor you on this medication.

TYPICAL DOSE: 2 mg to start, working up to an average dose of 2 mg twice a day, taken with food. Taking a one-month rest from the medication after six months is often recommended, though controversial, to try to prevent fibrosis. A substitute medication can be prescribed during that time.

SIDE EFFECTS: Nausea, hot feelings in the head, and leg cramps are common. Occasional severe gastrointestinal upset. "Feeling weird" is not unusual, although most people do not have significant side effects with methysergide.

3. NEURONTIN (GABAPENTIN)

Neurontin is very promising as an antipain and antiheadache medication. Like Depakote, it is also prescribed for seizures. Neurontin is one of the few medications that does not irritate the liver; it's proven to be very safe with few serious consequences, thus rendering it very useful for treating headache. It is one of the few newer preventive medications to come along, as most of the recent breakthroughs have been in abortive or "as-needed" medications, such as Imitrex, Zomig, Maxalt, Amerge, and Migranal. However, sedation, fatigue, and dizziness are relatively common.

TYPICAL DOSE: 300 mg once or twice per day to start, increasing as needed to as much as 2,400 mg per day. The average dose ranges from 900 mg to 2,000 mg per day. Neurontin is available in 100-mg, 300-mg, 400-mg, 600-mg, and 800-mg capsules, and is moderately expensive.

SIDE EFFECTS: Sedation or dizziness may occur. "Cognitive" side effects, such as difficulty thinking through problems, spaciness, mild confusion, and fatigue, can also occur, but most people tolerate Neurontin very well. Weight gain occasionally occurs.

4. NATURAL HERBS/SUPPLEMENTS FOR PREVENTING MIGRAINES (FEVERFEW, MAGNESIUM OXIDE, VITAMIN B₂; SEE ALSO CHAPTER 14)

- **FEVERFEW**

  Feverfew is an herb with the active ingredient parthenolide. As with other herbs, different farms will produce feverfew with widely different concentrations of parthenolide. This quality control remains a problem with herbs. The usual dose has been two or three capsules in the morning each day. Occasionally, feverfew is also used as an abortive to stop a headache in progress. Feverfew may also be ingested as a liquid (concentrated drops). In Europe, feverfew is often ingested by chewing the leaves that people grow in their backyards. Side effects tend to be mouth sores, or in rare circumstances, bleeding problems. Feverfew should not be used during pregnancy or if pregnancy may be a possibility.

- **MAGNESIUM OXIDE**

Magnesium oxide is readily available in pharmacies in doses from 250 mg to 400 mg. The usual dose is 250 mg to 500 mg once per day as a preventive. It has been demonstrated that magnesium levels are low in the brains of migraine sufferers. Gastrointestinal (stomach) side effects may limit its use. Do not take with calcium, as the magnesium will not be absorbed. Magnesium oxide may be useful for menstrual migraine. Long-term effects of magnesium supplements, if any, are not known.

- **VITAMIN B$_2$ (RIBOFLAVIN)**

Riboflavin, also known as Vitamin B$_2$, has been used as a daily preventive for migraine in the large dose of 400 mg per day. In at least two studies, riboflavin was found to be somewhat effective. However, long-term side effects of large doses of vitamin B$_2$ are not known.

THIRD-LINE MEDICATIONS FOR PREVENTING MIGRAINES

These third-line approaches to preventing migraines are usually the treatment of last resort. Doctors won't prescribe them until you have tried other options that have potentially fewer problems. Although all these treatments are used with caution, your doctor will take even greater precautions if you are over fifty.

QUICK REFERENCE GUIDE: THIRD-LINE
MEDICATIONS FOR PREVENTING MIGRAINES

1. MAO INHIBITORS

Powerful antidepressants that can prevent migraines, but insomnia and weight gain are common.

2. LONG-ACTING OPIOIDS (METHADONE, OXYCONTIN, KADIAN)

Effective for severe, refractive, chronic daily headaches and migraines. Sedation and constipation are common. Oxycontin and Kadian are particularly well tolerated.

3. STIMULANTS/AMPHETAMINES (RITALIN, PHENTERMINE, DEXTROAMPHETAMINE, METHAMPHETAMINE)

Sometimes useful as a last resort.

4. INTRAVENOUS DIHYDROERGOTAMINE (DHE)

Very safe and effective but requires going to see the doctor for office injections.

5. DAILY TRIPTANS (IMITREX, AMERGE, MAXALT, ZOMIG, RELPAX)

Expensive, and the possibility of long-term side effects make these a last resort.

1. MAO (MONOAMINE OXIDASE) INHIBITORS

These medications are helpful if you get severe migraines (or chronic daily headaches) and other medications haven't worked. They also can be very helpful to counter depression, anxiety, and panic attacks. These are powerful medications with very serious possible side effects.

Although MAO inhibitors may be used with relative safety and may be the only medications that will help prevent your migraines and daily headaches, it is essential that you avoid certain foods and medications while taking an MAO inhibitor because they could significantly increase the risk of a high blood pressure crisis. These include:

- Sumatriptan (Imitrex) or other triptans (Amerge, Maxalt, Zomig, Relpax)
- Meperidine (Demerol)
- Over-the-counter decongestants (Check with the doctor if you want to take any OTC medication.)
- Excessive caffeine (more than two cups of coffee or cola drinks), chocolate
- Red wine, sherry, ale, and beer
- Tenderized meats, liver, fermented meats (pepperoni, summer sausage, salami, bologna)
- Caviar, dried or salted fish, herring
- Aged cheeses
- Yogurt, sour cream
- Bananas, overripe figs, avocado, raisins
- Yeast extracts, soy sauce
- Fava beans

Occasionally, an MAO inhibitor is used in conjunction with certain other antidepressants, beta-blockers, and calcium blockers; if you take such a combination, your doctor will need to monitor you closely.

- **PHENELZINE (NARDIL)**
  This is the most effective and frequently used MAO inhibitor, but liver function and blood pressure need to be monitored with its use.

  TYPICAL DOSE: 15 mg to start, taken at night, and sometimes increased over one to three weeks to an average dose of 45 mg if needed. If ineffective even at 60 mg, then another medication should be tried instead. Take at night to avoid interactions with certain foods. If phenelzine causes insomnia, try taking it in the early morning.

  SIDE EFFECTS: Insomnia and weight gain. Less common side effects include a dry mouth, constipation, rapid heartbeat, agitation or other mood changes, swelling of the hands or feet.

2. Long-Acting Opioids (methadone, Oxycontin, MS Contin, Kadian)

For a tiny select group of severe headache sufferers with refractive chronic daily headaches and migraines, long-acting opioids can be useful. The short-acting ones, such as hydrocodone or codeine, tend to cause addiction and rebound headaches when used daily. If daily opioids are necessary, the longer-acting ones, which are effective for eight to sixteen hours, do not cause rebound headaches and may be used once or twice per day on a regular (but not on an "as-needed") basis. Doses need to be kept low with all of these medications. Oxycontin and Kadian are particularly well tolerated.

Another advantage of these opioids is that they do not cause the weight gain and other side effects that many other preventive medications do. However, these are an absolute last resort to be used when basically nothing else works. They may cause sedation, depression, and constipation. Although less than 5 percent of patients with pain or severe headaches who use narcotics ever become addicted, it's still a small risk but one that's definitely worth taking if other options don't work. Most people do become dependent on these medications, but not addicted, and that is a crucial difference (see the section in Chapter 5 on addiction versus dependence).

- **Methadone**
Methadone is inexpensive and used in low doses, 5 mg to 20 mg per day. It is crucial to begin with very low doses. If methadone is overused in the beginning, it is extremely dangerous.

- **Oxycontin**
Oxycontin is a long-acting form of oxycodone that is well tolerated and available in multiple doses. Again, doses must be kept low, 40 mg per day or less.

- **Kadian or MS Contin**
These are longer-acting forms of morphine. They are also useful because they are very long lasting (particularly Kadian). The usual dose of Kadian is 20 mg once or twice a day.

3. STIMULANTS (RITALIN, PHENTERMINE, DEXTROAMPHETAMINE)

Stimulants are occasionally useful as last-resort therapy. Occasionally these are used as an adjunct to long-acting opioids or other medications. Addiction, however, is always a concern with these medications. While some patients may respond well to stimulants as a last resort, they are only used when absolutely no other measures have been helpful.

4. INTRAVENOUS DIHYDROERGOTAMINE (IV DHE)

This treatment is very safe and extremely effective for preventing and relieving frequent or severe migraines, daily headaches, or cluster headaches, but its use requires going to a doctor's office or hospital to receive intravenous injections. Typically, IV DHE will give you good relief for at least one or two months, occasionally for as long as eight months.

Your doctor may also recommend this treatment if you have become dependent on narcotic painkillers, such as codeine, or analgesic overuse, and, as a result, you suffer from rebound headaches. This medication can help you withdraw from your dependence.

If you have high blood pressure, your doctor will treat you cautiously with the medication. If you have heart disease or peripheral vascular disease, your doctor probably won't use it at all.

TYPICAL DOSE: *When administered at the doctor's office,* the doctor will ask you to take an antinausea medication at home, preferably Reglan because it is mild, and a few Tums. At the office, you will get an injection, probably a shot twice a day for one to three days, or a total of two to six doses.

When administered at the hospital, the injection can be given three times in one day, or up to nine doses in three days. The accompanying antinausea medication can be stronger, so you can take larger doses, which, in turn, will be more sedating. Typically, you'll need a two- or three-day stay in the hospital, so the staff can monitor and care for you.

SIDE EFFECTS: Nausea, hot feeling in the head, a temporary tightness in the throat or chest, leg and muscle cramps, and a temporary rise in blood pressure. Occasional diarrhea or brief muscle tension headache afterward. The side effects, if present, usually last less than one hour. To combat nausea, which is common, an antinausea medication is usually taken before the DHE.

5. DAILY TRIPTANS (IMITREX, AMERGE, MAXALT, ZOMIG, RELPAX)

For some people with chronic daily headaches and frequent migraines, the only medication that is useful is a low dose of a triptan on a daily basis. Because these medications are relatively new, long-term side effects are still unknown. Because they are expensive and may produce long-term side effects, these medications are an absolute last resort. For some people with severe chronic daily headache and migraine, however, a daily triptan is the only effective measure.

CASE STUDIES

Here are examples of how this preventive information might be applied in a real situation.

CARLY

INITIAL VISIT: Carly, a twenty-two-year-old student, gets about one migraine every week. Her migraines started at age fourteen but have increased in the past year. Carly has asthma, but otherwise is healthy.

She tends to get more migraines around her menstrual period and with stress or weather changes. Red wine also gives her a migraine. Carly gets some relief from Excedrin or Fiorinal, but the headaches are severe, with nausea accompanying most of them. Carly's mother also get migraines.

With four severe migraines a month, Carly is on the borderline between needing daily preventive medication and treating the headaches once they begin. She is placed on naproxen, a nonsteroidal anti-inflammatory, once a day as a preventive medication. The NSAIDs have an advantage because they do not cause drowsiness or weight gain; however, they can irritate the stomach, liver, or kidneys. Carly is also given Imitrex Nasal Spray.

WEEK 6:   The migraines are down to two per month and the Imitrex works well, stopping the headache within one hour.

WEEK 12:   By this time, both medications seem to be losing their effectiveness, so Carly's doctor changes her daily preventive from naproxen to verapamil (Isoptin, Calan, Verelan), which does not affect Carly's asthma (a beta-blocker, such as Inderal, would affect the asthma). The sumatriptan is changed to Maxalt, to relieve a migraine when it occurs. The doctor also gives her Compazine capsules for nausea.

WEEK 16:   The verapamil is ineffective. Carly is getting at least four migraines a month. The Maxalt is partially effective, although it makes her feel somewhat tired; the Compazine helps decrease her nausea. Carly's doctor takes her off the verapamil as a preventive medication and gives her amitriptyline, an antidepressant that is widely used to prevent headaches. Depakote would also be considered.

WEEK 20:   Carly sleeps well with the amitriptyline because of its sedative effect, but the doses are kept low and she does not have a problem with daytime drowsiness. The headaches are down to one per month. Although the Maxalt is somewhat effective to relieve a migraine when it occurs, Carly also begins taking Fiorinal, either alone or with the Maxalt, to enhance pain relief.

THE FUTURE: As her condition and sensitivity to side effects shift, Carly's medication may change. Her doctor may take her off preventives altogether, or switch her to another preventive, perhaps Depakote or a different NSAID or antidepressant. There are also other abortives that may be more effective, such as Zomig, Amerge, Imitrex tablets or injections, Migranal (DHE) Nasal Spray, or the older ergotamines.

SALLY

INITIAL VISIT: Sally, a forty-year-old social worker, gets two migraines a week (more during her menstrual period) and is somewhat anxious and depressed. She has had headaches for many years, but they've gotten worse during the past year; she also suffers from asthma. Stress, weather, cigarette smoke, and missing a meal tend to trigger her migraines. When over-the-counter medications stopped relieving her pain, her general practitioner prescribed Midrin and Fiorinal, which helped a little. Because of the frequency of migraines and coexisting anxiety and depression, she had also been given the antidepressant amitriptyline as a daily preventive to take at night. She comes to her initial visit frustrated because she has gained weight and becomes excessively tired from the amitriptyline.

Sally is switched to Zoloft, with instructions to slowly increase the dose until she is taking 50 mg per day. She is also given Imitrex Nasal Spray and tablets; she will use the nasal spray for a fast-onset headache with nausea, and the tablets (if she can keep them down) for slow-onset headaches. Sally also keeps her Fiorinal as a backup for the pain. (Having two or three abortive medications or more is quite common, so patients can choose between different medications in different situations during their migraines.)

WEEK 6: The migraines are slightly, but not significantly, better with the Zoloft, but Sally experiences much less anxiety and depression. She is slightly fatigued from the Zoloft and has a mild problem with sweating, but she is more than willing to trade these conditions for the improvement in her anxiety and depression. The Imitrex Nasal Spray is not as effective as the tablets, and she wishes to try the injections. Sally is taught how to use the Imitrex auto-injector.

WEEK 12: Sally is still getting migraines about twice a week, but the Imitrex injections are very effective. However, Sally wants to try something new to reduce the number of migraines because they are significantly interfering with her life. She awakens with them at five or six A.M., and they leave her sleep-deprived all day. Her doctor adds Depakote, one of the first-line preventive medications, to the Zoloft. Sally is to take a low dose of Depakote, 250 mg twice a day.

WEEK 14: The Depakote is causing some weight gain, but it has decreased the headaches to twice a month, down from twice a week. Sally effectively uses Imitrex injections, and occasionally she uses the Imitrex tablets and Fiorinal as well.

THE FUTURE: Other preventive medications that would be useful for Sally include verapamil, NSAIDs, or Neurontin. If she continues to gain weight, the Depakote may be stopped and another preventive medication instituted. Alternatively, the doctor may simply see what happens after stopping the Depakote. Headache sufferers often go into a fluid situation with the preventive medications, going off and on them, switching, and increasing or decreasing doses (depending upon effectiveness and side effects). Alternative abortives, such as other triptans (Maxalt, Amerge, Zomig, Relpax), are possibilities for Sally in the future.

7

·········

WOMEN, HORMONES,
AND MIGRAINES

FLUCTUATING HORMONES, especially the progestins and estrogens, seem to play an important role in influencing migraines in women. At age ten, as many boys as girls suffer from migraines. By puberty, many girls who never before had migraine problems start having them, and by the midteens, migraines become much more common and more severe among girls than boys.

Puberty and the days around ovulation and menstruation are particularly vulnerable times for women who are susceptible to migraines. A woman's thirties and forties are commonly the worst decades, with the migraines becoming severe and prolonged. Many women experience relief during pregnancy and often after menopause. Birth control pills occasionally trigger, yet occasionally improve migraines, but for most women they don't exert much influence on the pattern of headaches.

Researchers aren't sure exactly why women's hormones affect migraines. In the 1970s, researchers thought that declining estrogen levels were a major reason behind migraines, but recent research paints a more complex picture. It's been found that the platelets and prostaglandins in the bloodstreams of women with hormonal headaches look different than those of women who are not suffering from these headaches. However, the major differences may actually occur in the brain, involving the center, called the hypothalamus, that controls the ovarian hormones. Indeed, the hypothalamus may be the ultimate source of the severe menstrual migraine. In any event, chances are that the tendency to get menstrual migraines is inherited.

MENSTRUAL MIGRAINES

Menstrual migraines can be especially miserable because they're often more severe and harder to treat than other kinds of migraines. Typically, they occur before, during, or after a woman's period. If you suffer from menstrual migraines, you may have headaches during ovulation and get migraines that aren't triggered by hormones at other times of the month as well. Menstrual migraines are a major reason for lost worktime, injured relationships, and reduced quality of life.

HORMONAL INFLUENCES

Researchers suspect that the hormone mechanisms, which are controlled by the brain, are somehow different in women who get hormonal, or menstrual, headaches than in other women, though consistent patterns haven't emerged. Some studies have found that women who get premenstrual migraines have higher levels of the hormones progestin and estrogen before their periods than women who don't get headaches. Others suggest that a drop in estrogen levels, which occurs just before a period (and after menopause or a hysterectomy), can trigger headaches (yet in other women this drop helps their migraines). Still other menstrual migraines may be related to the fluid build-up that occurs with menstruation.

Both estrogen and the progestin progesterone are known to influence serotonin receptors, and low levels of estrogen can significantly impact the hypothalamus (the gland that controls the hormonal secretion functions) and its control mechanisms. The truth is, researchers do not yet understand the mechanisms behind hormones and headaches.

TREATING MENSTRUAL MIGRAINES

Mild to moderate menstrual headaches that last only a day or so can often be relieved with one of the over-the-counter medications or anti-inflammatories discussed in Chapter 2, such as Excedrin, Aleve, ibuprofen, or a prescription NSAID.

Severe, prolonged menstrual migraines, which are not uncommon, can be relieved with injections and then prevented by following several approaches, as summarized below.

RELIEVING MENSTRUAL MIGRAINES: In general, your doctor will probably use the same strategies to relieve a menstrual migraine as a general migraine. When the migraines are severe, the cortisone medications, especially Decadron or prednisone, in limited amounts, are among the most effective treatments. The triptans (Imitrex, Amerge, Maxalt, Zomig, Relpax) are extremely important in combating menstrual migraines. Many women need to resort to Imitrex injections, which are probably the most effective "as-needed" medication. If these strategies fail, a strong narcotic taken with a strong antinausea medication, such as Compazine, can help. Because menstrual migraines can be severe, many women must resort to these powerful treatments. Refer to Chapter 5 for detailed discussions of these medications.

PREVENTING MENSTRUAL MIGRAINES: As with general migraines, your menstrual migraines may be triggered by typical migraine foods, as outlined in Chapter 6. However, you may be sensitive to these foods only the week or so before your periods. To prevent menstrual migraines, experiment with abstaining from alcohol (especially red wine), chocolate, aged cheese, and other common migraine-trigger foods; eating regularly and including plenty of complex carbohydrates (pasta, rice, beans, whole grains) to maintain steady levels of blood sugar; exercising; and using relaxation techniques to minimize stress. Also, experiment with caffeine — in some women, caffeine helps; in others, it is a trigger.

If your menstrual migraines are predictable, moderately severe, and not responsive to nonmedication strategies, your doctor may suggest trying preventive medication beginning on the day before the expected onset of the migraine and continuing until two to three days past the time you normally get migraines. Details on medications doctors typically use for preventing menstrual migraines follow. *Note: Many of the medications mentioned in this chapter have been discussed in detail in previous chapters. Please check the index to locate more detailed information.*

MEDICATIONS FOR PREVENTING
MENSTRUAL MIGRAINES

**QUICK REFERENCE GUIDE: MEDICATIONS FOR
PREVENTING MENSTRUAL MIGRAINES**

**1. NSAIDs (NAPROXEN, IBUPROFEN, FLURBIPROFEN,
MECLOFENAMATE SODIUM)**

The backbone of menstrual migraine therapy: effective, well tolerated. Start three days prior to the expected onset. Gastrointestinal upset is common. Doctors do not yet know if the newer NSAIDs, which are easier on the stomach, such as Vioxx, will be effective for menstrual migraine.

**2. ERGOTAMINE DERIVATIVES (ERGOTAMINE TARTRATE
[ERGOMAR], ERGONOVINE [ERGOTRATE], DHE)**

Start one to three days prior to onset. These drugs can be effective but often cause gastrointestinal upset and nausea, and can trigger rebound headaches.

**3. DIURETICS (DYAZIDE, HYDROCHLOROTHIAZIDE,
MODURETIC)**

Water pills that are occasionally useful.

**4. HORMONAL APPROACHES (TAMOXIFEN [NOLVADEX],
ESTROGEN, CONTINUOUS BIRTH CONTROL PILLS)**

These have potential risks and side effects such as nausea, bleeding, weight gain, and edema.

**5. TRIPTANS (AMERGE, IMITREX, MAXALT, ZOMIG,
RELPAX)**

For some women, these are the most effective abortive and preventive therapy.

**1. NONSTEROIDAL ANTI-INFLAMMATORIES (NSAIDs)
(NAPROXEN, IBUPROFEN, FLURBIPROFEN, KETOPROFEN)**
Anti-inflammatories are the backbone of preventive therapy for

menstrual migraines because they have the fewest side effects and are well tolerated. When one NSAID doesn't work, your doctor will often suggest trying another before progressing to a different class of medication.

TYPICAL DOSE: Take three days before expected headache and continue until several days past the expected time. Timing can be tricky. For ibuprofen, from 400 mg to 2,400 mg per day, split up during day. For naproxen, 500 mg, once or twice a day. For flurbiprofen (Ansaid), 100 mg twice a day.

SIDE EFFECTS: Stomach upset, stomach pain, heartburn. Stop the NSAID if you experience more than mild stomach problems from it.

2. Ergotamine Derivatives

These medications are often effective, although they do carry a risk for triggering rebound headaches.

- **Ergotamine tartrate (Ergomar)**
  TYPICAL DOSE: Usually 2 mg of ergotamine per day.
  SIDE EFFECTS: In addition to rebound headaches, ergotamine derivatives may cause nausea or severe gastrointestinal upset, as well as nervousness and leg cramps.
- **Ergonovine (Ergotrate)**
  This medication is well tolerated and occasionally effective.
  TYPICAL DOSE: 0.2 mg, two to four times a day.
  SIDE EFFECTS: Same as the other ergotamines, though usually milder.
- **Dihydroergotamine (DHE)**
  This medication is either injected or taken as a nasal spray (Migranal) that is very convenient. DHE is usually very well tolerated.
  TYPICAL DOSE: 1 mg a day.
  SIDE EFFECTS: Nausea, harmless throat or chest tightness, mild muscle contraction, leg cramps, a hot feeling about the head.

3. DIURETICS
HYDROCHLOROTHIAZIDE (DYAZIDE, MODURETIC)

Diuretics, also known as water pills, are only occasionally helpful for migraines but also help other menstrual symptoms, such as bloating. They are generally well tolerated, but even though they are used for only a short time during the month, care must be taken to avoid losing too much potassium. Diuretics should be taken only under a doctor's care.

TYPICAL DOSE: Half a pill or one pill taken in the morning for two to three days prior to and with the menstrual period.

SIDE EFFECTS: Frequent urination. Occasional rashes, weakness, or dizziness.

4. HORMONAL APPROACHES

If your menstrual migraines are very severe and debilitating, your doctor may recommend a stronger approach, such as hormonal therapy. Before trying these powerful drugs, though, be sure you are well informed of the potential risks. They often have unpleasant side effects, which you'll have to weigh against the pain and degraded quality of life you suffer from headaches.

- #### TAMOXIFEN (NOLVADEX)

  One of the more effective menstrual migraine preventives, this medication is otherwise used in breast cancer therapy and prevention. It sometimes decreases the frequency and severity of migraines and daily headaches that occur at other times of the month as well.

  TYPICAL DOSE: 10 mg (the range is 5 mg to 20 mg) each day for seven to fourteen days, starting one to two weeks prior to menstruation.

  SIDE EFFECTS: Occasional and mild nausea, hot flashes, and menstrual irregularities; infrequent rashes, vaginal bleeding, vaginal discharges, weight gain, edema, headaches, shortness of breath, loss of appetite, pain in the legs, blurred vision, and dizziness. In very large doses in animals, malignant liver tumors have been reported. Frequent Pap smears are necessary to assess any signs of early cervical cancer.

- **ESTROGEN**

If your migraines are severe, prolonged, and generally debilitating, they may warrant using a strong medication. Estrogen sometimes works to prevent menstrual migraines that are triggered by the estrogen decrease that occurs during the late luteal phase of the menstrual cycle. In some women, however, estrogen exacerbates headaches.

TYPICAL DOSE: 0.05 mg of ethinyl estradiol (Estinyl) each day for five days before menses and continued for two days after flow. Or 1 or 2 mg of micronized estradiol (Estrace) each day with same regimen. Or an estrogen skin patch (Estraderm) changed twice weekly and used for a total of seven days.

SIDE EFFECTS: Estrogen carries many potential side effects, including breakthrough bleeding, irregular or suspended periods, menstrual flow changes, endometrial hyperplasia, yeast infection (vaginal candidiasis), nausea, abdominal cramps, colitis or cholestatic jaundice, hair loss (alopecia) or abnormal hair growth (hirsutism), hives, headache, dizziness, depression, weight gain or loss, edema, decreased libido, and tenderness of the breasts. Long-term use may also increase the risk of endometrial cancer and breast cancer.

- **CONTINUOUS BIRTH CONTROL PILLS**

For some women with extremely severe, prolonged menstrual migraine, low-dose continuous (noncycling) birth control pills can help. Women can use birth control pills for a number of months, to relieve the devastating headaches for that period of time. This approach is relatively safe and at times is the only effective therapy. While birth control pills may help decrease headaches, when they are used on a cyclical basis (in the usual manner), menstrual migraines are often more severe. A few of the newer pills (such as Mircette) continue to deliver a tiny amount of estrogen even during the menstrual period; these may be better than the older kinds for menstrual migraine. Women who smoke cigarettes, however, should not take the birth control pill. While this link has not been conclusively proven, the birth control pill may slightly raise the risk of stroke in women with migraines.

- **OOPHORECTOMY (REMOVING THE OVARIES)**
In very rare circumstances, some women who are over forty and suffer from prolonged, severe, refractive menstrual migraines find relief with Lupron injections to stop the menstrual cycle. When this approach works, a few women have had an oophorectomy to relieve the devastating headaches permanently. This step is controversial, and there's no consensus whether it is ever indicated or appropriate.

5. TRIPTANS (IMITREX, AMERGE, MAXALT, ZOMIG, RELPAX)

For some women, triptans are the most effective abortive and preventive therapy. Ideally, the longer-acting one (Amerge) may be best; however, Imitrex effectively prevents menstrual headaches in certain women.

TYPICAL DOSE: The usual dose is one tablet twice per day, starting about one day prior to the "usual" onset of the migraine. These usually would be continued for three to five days. The timing of a menstrual migraine is often difficult to predict, however. Amerge (2.5 mg) is very well tolerated and is particularly suited to this use. The FDA, however, has not yet indicated triptans for this use. (See Chapter 5 for a complete discussion on triptans.)

6. VITAMINS AND MINERALS (SEE CHAPTER 14)

Magnesium oxide (250 mg to 500 mg per day) has been helpful for some women with menstrual migraines. It is usually taken daily, or for one week prior to and with the menstrual period. Long-term side effects, if any, are not known.

Calcium may be helpful as well (750 mg to 1500 mg daily). In addition, Vitamin B_2 (riboflavin), 400 mg per day, has been superior to a placebo for migraine prevention in several studies. Long-term side effects, if any, are not known.

HEADACHES DURING PREGNANCY

If you suffer from migraines, chances are that pregnancy, especially the second and third trimesters, will bring a welcome relief. If you do get headaches at this time, however, they are particularly hard to treat because you must avoid drugs that may potentially be harmful to the fetus. First try ice packs, relaxation therapy, and rest in a dark room. Ask your doctor about using small amounts of medication, such as acetaminophen (Tylenol). While caffeine decreases headaches, its use during pregnancy remains controversial. Limited amounts are probably fine. If you need something stronger, the doctor may try small doses of meperidine (Demerol), hydrocodone (Vicodin), or acetaminophen with codeine. Limited amounts of cortisone are also used on occasion. Take antinausea medications only if absolutely necessary, and only in small amounts. Over-the-counter preparations that may help nausea include Vitamin B_6 and Emetrol. For more severe nausea, Reglan or Compazine are occasionally used.

If your migraines are frequent and severe, or you get daily headaches that are intolerable, your doctor may recommend preventive medications with minimal doses after the first trimester. A beta-blocker (such as propranolol, metoprolol, nadolol, or timolol) is often prescribed and discontinued three weeks before delivery to avoid harming the baby. Be sure you understand all the risks before trying any of these medications.

When beta-blockers don't work or can't be used, the doctor may recommend a very low dose (such as 10 or 25 mg) of amitriptyline if daily preventive medication is necessary. However, there have been isolated reports that amitriptyline may trigger abnormalities in babies' arms or legs. Again, be sure you understand whatever risks that this or other medications pose during pregnancy. Prozac and Zoloft have been used during pregnancy, and preliminary studies indicate that they are probably safe. However, this has not been proven. You need to be completely informed about all the possible risks of any medications used during pregnancy.

HEADACHES DURING BREASTFEEDING

Like pregnant women, women who are breastfeeding should minimize taking medication. If they get headaches that require medications, they may take, as needed, acetaminophen, caffeine, and NSAIDs. If necessary, they may also take a narcotic painkiller. Because of sedation, Fioricet or Esgic are used with caution. Antihistamines are not used. Prochlorperazine (Compazine) is the antinausea drug of choice. Ergots and triptans are best avoided. Preventively, beta-blockers, calcium blockers, and Depakote can be used. Women may take steroids in limited situations for limited periods of time. Antidepressants are utilized with caution, although the SSRIs (selective serotonin reuptake inhibitors, such as Prozac, Zoloft, and Paxil) have been widely used during this period.

MIGRAINES DURING AND AFTER MENOPAUSE

Typically, migraines worsen during menopause, but then may improve afterward. Yet it is not uncommon to have a different experience: some women get worse headaches after menopause; others enjoy a complete cessation of head pain. Some women who have never had a headache problem get severe migraines for the first time during menopause. Still other women experience no change in their migraine patterns.

If possible, doctors generally minimize hormone replacement in migraine treatment. Although hormones seem to help some women, they worsen headaches more often than help them. For many women, hormones don't affect the headaches one way or another. If you take hormones for other reasons and want to reap the benefits of these hormones, talk to your doctor about whether they seem to affect your headaches. If your headaches become severe after taking hormones, it may be necessary to stop taking them.

Which hormones you take and how you use them can influence your headaches. In general, the natural estrogens, such as Premarin, tend to aggravate headaches more than the "synthetic estrogens," such as Estinyl and Estrace, do. The hormone patch, which delivers a smooth, controlled amount of estrogen, sometimes leads to fewer headaches. If you haven't had a hysterectomy, progestins (progesterone, such as Provera), along with the estrogen, are usually necessary. There are tablets that contain a combination of estrogen plus progesterone. Progestins often exacerbate headaches, and doctors prefer to minimize the progesterone. After a hysterectomy, the primary use of progestins (to prevent uterine cancer) is no longer necessary. Thus, after a hysterectomy, doctors often skip the progesterone.

Ideally, estrogens that are used continuously (noncycling) are better for headaches. When the estrogen is stopped for one week, the dip in estrogen levels may increase headaches. However, by using continuous estrogen, the risk for breast or uterine cancer may be slightly increased. After a hysterectomy, women are often placed on continuous estrogen without a break.

The "as-needed" and preventive medications basically remain the same during and after menopause. However, as you get older, you become at higher risk for cardiac (heart) problems, and so doctors may recommend that you abstain from using the triptans (Imitrex, Amerge, Maxalt, Zomig, Relpax). Ergotamines are rarely used after age fifty. As for preventive medication, weight gain is often a major problem during these years. Searching for preventive medication that does not exacerbate or cause weight gain is important. The preventive medications that tend to minimize weight gain include NSAIDs, calcium blockers, and select antidepressants, such as Vivactil, Prozac, Zoloft, Paxil, Celexa, Wellbutrin, and Effexor.

CASE STUDY

Here is a fairly typical case of a woman who gets menstrual migraines and how her doctor helps her manage them.

SUZY

INITIAL VISIT: Suzy, a thirty-four-year-old social worker and mother of two children, gets severe migraines for four days each month, usually beginning one day before her menstrual period. She has regular periods, every twenty-eight days, and no other health problems. She has tried, with little or no benefit, ibuprofen, Fiorinal, Midrin, Tylenol 3, Vicodin, and Excedrin.

Because Suzy usually begins sensing the migraine just prior to the beginning of her period, she is advised to start naproxen, an NSAID, three days before her menstrual period. Naproxen is particularly effective in preventing menstrual migraines. For an abortive medication, the doctor prescribes sumatriptan (Imitrex) tablets because Suzy does not want to give herself injections at this time.

WEEK 16: Suzy reports that the naproxen helped for the first two months, but then lost its effectiveness. The Imitrex tablets do not help much. Suzy's doctor prescribes flurbiprofen (Ansaid), another NSAID, as a preventive medication, Imitrex injections and a small dose of dexamethasone (Decadron) as an abortive medication.

WEEK 24: Suzy says the flurbiprofen was not effective and because she gets incapacitating and prolonged (four days) migraine attacks, she is prepared to try hormonal therapy to prevent them. She and her doctor discuss fully the risks and possible side effects, from nausea, hot flashes, and rashes to vaginal discharges, weight gain, and shortness of breath. Suzy receives a prescription for estrogen to take before her periods to prevent the attacks. Her abortive regimen is working in that it shortens her attacks significantly.

WEEK 32: The estrogen is not effective, so Suzy's doctor prescribes tamoxifen (Nolvadex) to take for one week before menstrual periods.

WEEK 40: Suzy reports that the tamoxifen is working well and that she feels in good control. When she does get a migraine, the Imitrex injections and dexamethasone usually help.

THE FUTURE: Other possibilities as preventive approaches include: low-dose (continuous) birth control pills, water pills (diuretics) used prior to the menstrual period, or triptans (Imitrex, Amerge, Maxalt, Zomig, Relpax) used for four or five days. As-needed ergotamines, strong narcotics, injections of Toradol (injected by Suzy at home) or Stadol Nasal Spray are additional possibilities.

8

· · · · · · · ·

TREATING TENSION
HEADACHES IN PROGRESS

MIGRAINES may be the most common headaches treated by doctors, but tension headaches plague the general population much more commonly; more than three-quarters of all headaches are tension headaches. Although the name "tension headache" may seem to imply that all headaches come from stress and tension, these are *not* psychological problems. This name is actually very misleading.

WHAT IS A TENSION HEADACHE?

Tension headaches can hurt anywhere around the head, but usually they cause pain on both sides. Sufferers often describe them as band-like, aching, pressing, tightening, or dull. Some people wake up in the early morning with the headache pounding or throbbing. Although usually mild or moderate, these headaches can be severe, waxing and waning throughout the day.

Unlike migraines, these milder headaches come on with no warning or auras, but most people can go on coping with work or home responsibilities. When tension headaches are severe, however, they may be accompanied by dizziness, nausea, and sensitivity to bright lights, much like migraines. Because it is sometimes difficult to distinguish between a severe tension headache and a mild migraine, many researchers suspect that the two headaches are the same illness, with tension headaches at the milder end of the spectrum.

Tension headaches may start at any age; about 40 percent of people start getting them in childhood or in their teens. Whether they will continue for a lifetime is unpredictable. Almost 40 percent of children and adolescents with tension headaches do outgrow their headaches by age twenty. However, if a child has had daily headaches for several years and has a parent who has had migraines or daily headaches, the child is likely to have them for years as well, although they may stop for months or even years, and then recur. In adults who get migraines and tension headaches, the migraines usually decline after age fifty but the tension headache pattern often persists.

TYPES OF TENSION HEADACHES

Usually tension headaches occur periodically, and in most cases, an over-the-counter pain reliever, a nap, and a relaxation exercise will relieve them. Ice packs applied to the head may also help.

When they occur more frequently, though, they are either *episodic,* occurring at least twice a week, but not more than fifteen times a month, or *chronic* or *daily,* occurring more than fifteen days a month for at least six months, or almost every day. The lines between the two get blurry if you get spells of daily tension headaches for weeks or months, and then very few headaches for a period of time. Also, many people who get tension headaches get migraines from time to time. For some people, the daily tension headache is much more of a problem than the occasional migraine; other people don't mind the daily headaches but are compelled to do something about their migraines. You are certainly not alone if you suffer from these frequent headaches — more than five million people in the United States get moderate or severe chronic daily headaches.

TENSION HEADACHES: NOT PSYCHOLOGICAL BUT INHERITED

Just like migraine headaches, tension headaches are not psychological or "all in the head" but legitimate medical illnesses. Although stress and tension trigger the headaches or make them worse, they are not the true cause of the pain. In fact, the term "tension headache" is erroneous and promotes this misconception. That is why many doctors call these headaches "muscle contraction headaches" instead. As with migraines, the real root of the headache, or cause, is a genetically inherited predisposition to triggers that produce increased muscular tension and changes in blood vessels and the central nervous system. The triggers may be stress, daily hassles, anxiety, or other factors, such as missing a meal, bright lights, undersleeping, and cigarette smoke.

Researchers suspect that tension headaches, like migraines, are caused by serotonin changes in the brain. In many ways, tension headaches and migraines are related.

- Both respond to similar medications: antidepressants, calcium blockers, anti-inflammatories, and beta-blockers.
- Both are linked to similar biochemical changes.
- Both are commonly associated with neck pain and muscle spasm.
- Both are often linked to a family history of headaches.
- Both commonly involve muscle tenderness on the head and brain blood flow changes.
- A mild migraine is very difficult to distinguish from a severe tension headache.
- The vast majority of people with chronic daily headaches also get migraines.

TREATMENT FOR TENSION HEADACHES

When the occasional tension headache occurs, the correct way to treat it is very similar to the suggestions offered in Chapter 2.

- Use a relaxation technique.
- Apply ice to your head.
- Try to ignore the pain if it is mild.
- Consider taking medication.

As always, the goal is to take as little medication as possible. If you need medication, your doctor will probably begin by suggesting a first-line abortive. These medications can be very effective, but if overused they carry the risk of causing rebound headaches. If you take numerous pills on a daily basis — more than two or three a day — you need to use relaxation methods more regularly or consider trying preventive medication.

All these medications are discussed in detail in Chapters 2, 5, and 6. We present them here in order of preference for tension headaches, and review their most salient features.

FIRST-LINE MEDICATIONS FOR ABORTING TENSION HEADACHES

QUICK REFERENCE GUIDE: FIRST-LINE MEDICATIONS FOR RELIEVING TENSION HEADACHES

1. ACETAMINOPHEN (TYLENOL), ASPIRIN
   OTC pain relief. Acetaminophen is very well tolerated but much less effective than other treatments. Aspirin often upsets stomach. Can cause rebound headaches if used too much.

2. NAPROXEN (ANAPROX DS, ALEVE)
   OTC, effective, but gastrointestinal upset is common.

3. IBUPROFEN (MOTRIN, ADVIL, NUPRIN, RUFEN, HALTRAN, IBUPRIN, MEDIPREN, MIDOL 200, TRENDAR)

OTC, effective, but gastrointestinal upset is common; however, ibuprofen is more effective for headache than acetaminophen.

4. CAFFEINE

OTC caffeine beverages or tablets make other medications more effective and reduce drowsiness. Too much can cause rebound headaches.

5. CAFFEINE-ASPIRIN COMBINATIONS (EXCEDRIN MIGRAINE, ANACIN, EXCEDRIN EXTRA-STRENGTH)

OTC, quite effective, but if used too often, cause rebound headaches. Excedrin has been a mainstay of headache therapy for many years.

6. KETOPROFEN (ORUDISKT, KETOPROFEN)

OTC NSAID; effective but often causes stomach upset.

7. MIDRIN

Effective, safe, mild, nonaddicting sedative. Fatigue and lightheadedness are common.

8. NORGESIC FORTE

Effective, quite strong, but gastrointestinal upset and fatigue are common.

9. VIOXX

A new NSAID with much less tendency to cause stomach bleeding.

1. ACETAMINOPHEN

Although less effective than aspirin or the medications that follow, acetaminophen is more easily tolerated. If you take more than 1,500 mg a day on a daily basis, rebound headaches may occur and you should consider daily preventive medication. (See Chapter 2.) Long-term daily use may lead to liver or kidney problems.

ASPIRIN

Aspirin is more effective than acetaminophen but has a greater risk of side effects. The main problems with aspirin are stomach irritation (gastritis or ulcers) and an increased tendency to bleed. Taking aspirin every day, however, has a number of beneficial effects, including decreased risk of heart attack, stroke, colon cancer, and perhaps Alzheimer's disease as well. (See Chapter 2.)

2. NAPROXEN (ALEVE)

The OTC version of naproxen is a very effective anti-inflammatory but can commonly cause stomach upset and nausea. (See Chapter 2.) Naproxen is longer-acting than ibuprofen; taking small amounts of caffeine may increase its effect.

3. IBUPROFEN (MOTRIN, ADVIL, NUPRIN, RUFEN, HALTRAN, IBUPRIN, MEDIPREN, MIDOL 200, TRENDAR)

Ibuprofen is also more effective than acetaminophen but may not be more effective than aspirin; stomach upset is relatively common. (See Chapter 2.) Taking small amounts of caffeine may help.

4. CAFFEINE

Taking caffeine, in coffee, soda, or pill form, can be very helpful. It may be taken individually or with a pain reliever to enhance its effectiveness. Caffeine overuse can also lead to rebound headaches. (See Chapter 2 for amounts of caffeine in foods and drinks.)

5. CAFFEINE-ASPIRIN COMBINATIONS

By combining the effects of caffeine with the pain relief of aspirin, these OTC products, such as Excedrin Extra-Strength, Excedrin Migraine, or Anacin, can be very effective, and have been a mainstay of OTC headache medication for years. (See Chapter 2.)

6. KETOPROFEN (OTC AS ORUDISKT, KETOPROFEN)

This well-tolerated anti-inflammatory is available over the counter in a low (12.5-mg) dose. The usual dose is two to four tablets every four to six hours, as needed. It may cause stomach upset or pain. Prescription ketoprofen is available in 50-mg and 75-mg doses, or as the long-acting Oruvail (100 mg, 150 mg, 200 mg). Taking small amounts of caffeine may enhance its effect. As with all NSAIDs, bleeding from the stomach or stomach ulcers may occur (particularly with frequent use).

7. MIDRIN

Midrin, a combination of a blood vessel constrictor, mild non-addicting sedative, and acetaminophen, is effective, safe, and well tolerated. Fatigue and lightheadedness are fairly common. By prescription only. (See Chapter 5.)

8. NORGESIC FORTE

Norgesic Forte, a combination of aspirin, caffeine, and a non-addicting muscle relaxant, is one of the strongest nonaddicting abortive medications for tension (and migraine) headaches, but gastrointestinal upset and fatigue are common. (See Chapter 5.)

9. VIOXX

Vioxx is a new anti-inflammatory that does not cause the stomach pain, ulcers, or bleeding that the other NSAIDs commonly do. Vioxx is available in 12.5-, 25-, and 50-mg tablets for acute pain; 50 mg may be used in a day, but for daily use, 25 mg is the maximum. While their safety has not completely been established, these newer NSAIDs are an exciting addition to the arsenal of headache medications.

SECOND-LINE MEDICATIONS FOR
ABORTING TENSION HEADACHES

If the first-line abortives don't work, your doctor may suggest stronger therapy with a more powerful pain reliever. These medications, which are potentially addicting, include the butalbital compounds (first-line migraine abortives), the narcotics (second-line migraine abortives), or the benzodiazepines (also second-line migraine abortives). If you take them once a week or less, these medications don't pose a problem. If you need them almost daily, they can be habit-forming and you should try preventive medication.

In rare circumstances — when first-line abortives, relaxation therapy, and preventive medications fail or cause too many side effects, and you and your doctor are confident that you would never use the medication to get high or lift you out of the dumps — your doctor may suggest using limited amounts of these habit-forming medications on a daily basis. We discuss all of these medications in more detail in Chapter 5, and we present them here in slightly different order for tension headaches.

(See Chapter 5 as well for a discussion of addiction versus dependency. The difference between the two is important to understand.)

QUICK REFERENCE GUIDE: SECOND-LINE MEDICATIONS FOR RELIEVING TENSION HEADACHES

1. **BUTALBITAL COMPOUNDS (FIORINAL, ESGIC, ESGIC PLUS, FIORICET, AND PHRENILIN)**

   Effective but habit-forming. Sedation or euphoria is common.

2. **NARCOTICS (CODEINE, HYDROCODONE, AND PROPOXYPHENE [DARVON, DARVOCET])**

   A last resort, needs to be limited per month; sedation, nausea, euphoria, constipation, dizziness, and itching fairly common.

3. **ULTRAM**

   Mild painkiller, but sometimes effective. Nausea and fatigue are fairly common.

4. **SEDATIVES (BENZODIAZEPINES: DIAZEPAM [VALIUM], CLONAZEPAM [KLONOPIN], CHLORDIAZEPOXIDE [LIBRIUM])**

   Sedation is common, must be monitored, a last resort; potentially habit-forming.

5. TRIPTANS (IMITREX, AMERGE, ZOMIG, MAXALT, RELPAX)
Though usually less useful for tension headaches, sometimes helpful for severe tension headaches. Many people find that their tension headaches do respond to low doses of a triptan.

1. BUTALBITAL COMPOUNDS (FIORINAL, ESGIC, ESGIC PLUS, FIORICET, PHRENILIN)

These are effective but habit-forming medications that should be used no more than once or twice a day. Sedation or euphoria are common. The generic form may not work as well as the brand name. Strict daily and monthly limits need to be set. (See Chapter 5.)

2. NARCOTICS: CODEINE, HYDROCODONE (VICODIN), PROPOXYPHENE (DARVON, DARVOCET)

These are last-resort medications that are generally not to be used daily and should have strict monthly limits. Your doctor will recommend them only if the milder abortives and daily preventive medications have not worked and your quality of life is significantly compromised by your tension headaches. Side effects may include, among others, sedation, nausea, euphoria, constipation, dizziness, and itching (or a rash, if you're allergic). (See Chapter 5.)

3. TRAMADOL (ULTRAM)

This excellent milder painkiller occasionally is useful for migraine sufferers. Tramadol may cause nausea or fatigue, but is generally well tolerated. The usual dose is one or two every four to six hours as needed. While addiction has occurred with Ultram, it is less likely than with the other narcotics.

4. SEDATIVES: BENZODIAZEPINES, SUCH AS DIAZEPAM (VALIUM) AND CLONAZEPAM (KLONOPIN) AND CHLORDIAZEPOXIDE (LIBRIUM)

These are habit-forming medications that commonly cause sedation. Your doctor should give you a monthly limit and monitor your use; if you need more than the limit, your doctor should switch your medication. If possible, avoid daily use. (See Chapter 5.)

5. TRIPTANS (IMITREX, ZOMIG, MAXALT, AMERGE, RELPAX)

These are generally thought of as "pure migraine" medications. However, severe tension headaches and milder migraines may share similar mechanisms in the brain. For many people, a small dose (half of one tablet) of a triptan may stop the tension headache. (See Chapter 5.)

If these medications fail or you take them too often, and you still suffer from severe and frequent daily headaches and feel that your quality of life is seriously compromised by these headaches, your doctor will probably discuss taking preventive medication as well as abortive medication. We discuss this strategy in the next chapter.

9

. . . .

PREVENTING TENSION HEADACHES

IF YOU'VE TRIED relaxation methods, small to moderate doses of the abortive medications, or are using these medications so often that you're running the risk of getting rebound headaches, don't despair. If your quality of life is still significantly impaired by the frequency and severity of your headaches, preventive medication may be the next step. Many people who switch to preventive medications find that they end up taking less medication and less powerful medication for better relief.

When considering preventive medications, keep in mind the guidelines discussed in Chapter 6.

1. Realize that the goal is moderate improvement with minimal side effects.
2. Be willing to change medications.
3. Try to be tolerant of mildly annoying side effects.
4. Be patient. Many medications take several weeks to become fully effective.
5. Be well informed about each drug you try.

CHOOSING PREVENTIVE MEDICATION

As with other headache situations, finding the right drug to prevent your daily chronic headaches isn't as simple as one would like. You and your doctor will have to consider many factors, such as whether you also get migraines, and your sleeping patterns and stomach sensitivity. As in other headache cases, chances are you'll need to take a trial-and-error approach, trying several different medications before you find the right balance of good pain relief with minimal side effects. Again, keep in mind that your goal is to improve your pain by at least 50 to 90 percent with as little medicine as possible. Your doctor will strongly consider whether you have a tendency toward anxiety or depression when choosing a preventive medication.

Many of the medications discussed in this chapter are not specifically indicated for headache by the Food and Drug Administration, as explained in Chapter 1. However, they are commonly used, and many doctors and patients have found them helpful. As with our other discussions of medications, this information is meant to serve as a guide only, and you should be sure to check the package insert for complete information about side effects and contraindications.

FIRST-LINE MEDICATIONS FOR PREVENTING TENSION HEADACHES

QUICK REFERENCE GUIDE: FIRST-LINE MEDICATIONS FOR PREVENTING TENSION HEADACHES

1. **DEPAKOTE**
   Quite effective, though gastrointestinal upset, fatigue, and weight gain may occur.
2. **ANTIDEPRESSANTS**
   Effective, but sedation, dizziness, a dry mouth, weight gain, and constipation are common.
3. **NONSTEROIDAL ANTI-INFLAMMATORIES (NSAIDS)**
   Less effective than antidepressants but without their side effects; however, GI upset is common. Long-term use may lead to stomach ulcers.

1. VALPROATE (DEPAKOTE)

A seizure medication, valproate, or Depakote, has become increasingly popular in headache treatment. However, it commonly causes gastrointestinal upset, fatigue, and weight gain; hair loss (alopecia) may also occur. (See Chapter 6 for a full discussion.)

2. ANTIDEPRESSANTS

These medications are the mainstay therapy for preventing daily headaches and may help whether you are depressed or not. Choosing an antidepressant depends on your anxiety level, age, sleeping patterns, and your tendency to become constipated. Although these medications may also help with depression, they are used here because they benefit headaches, most likely through a serotonin mechanism.

To compare these medications, see the table "The Antidepressants: Comparing Side Effects" and the more complete descriptions with typical dosages in Chapter 6. Here's a quick review of their main differences.

- **AMITRIPTYLINE (ELAVIL)**
  Effective for migraines and daily headaches, amitriptyline is inexpensive and can relieve insomnia. Unfortunately, a lot of people can't tolerate its side effects. Very low doses (10 mg at night) may be enough to help.
  SIDE EFFECTS: Sedation, dizziness, a dry mouth, weight gain, and constipation.

- **FLUOXETINE (PROZAC), SERTRALINE (ZOLOFT), OR PAROXETINE (PAXIL)**
  All of these medications, which are very similar, pose fewer side effects than amitriptyline, but they are not always as effective for headaches and are more expensive. They are good choices for people who suffer from the blues, a chronic, low-level depression, or for those over fifty, who need a medication with milder side effects. These are generally very safe medications; for headaches, low doses are used. (For more details on these medications, see Chapter 6.)
  SIDE EFFECTS: Nausea, anxiety, insomnia, and occasional

fatigue. Lack of weight gain (usually) and lack of sedation are major advantages. Reduced sexual desire is common.

- **PROTRIPTYLINE (VIVACTIL)**

Protriptyline is often used when daily headaches are also a problem. It is nonsedating and does not cause weight gain but is not as effective as amitriptyline.

SIDE EFFECTS: A dry mouth, constipation, and dizziness. Nervousness, insomnia, which can be countered by taking it in the morning, and, less often, blurred vision and stomach upset.

- **NORTRIPTYLINE (PAMELOR, AVENTYL)**

Although better tolerated than amitriptyline, nortriptyline is somewhat less effective. Often nortriptyline is a first-choice headache preventive for children, adolescents, and the elderly because its side effects are milder. Occasionally helpful for migraines, nortriptyline is usually more effective for chronic daily headache.

SIDE EFFECTS: Similar to amitriptyline but less severe, including sedation (which decreases over time), weight gain, a dry mouth, constipation, and dizziness.

- **DOXEPIN (SINEQUAN)**

Very similar to amitriptyline, doxepin is more effective than nortriptyline but has stronger side effects.

SIDE EFFECTS: Sedation, a dry mouth, weight gain, and constipation.

- **DESIPRAMINE (NORPRAMIN)**

Unlike amitriptyline, fluoxetine, protriptyline, and doxepin, desipramine is not generally useful for migraines but often helps chronic daily headaches. It's very well tolerated but generally not as effective as the other antidepressants. It is sometimes a first choice, however, for people over fifty who might be more sensitive to the antidepressants' side effects.

SIDE EFFECTS: Sleep disturbances if taken at night; other side effects are similar to amitriptyline but much milder.

- **TRIMIPRAMINE (SURMONTIL)**

This is a good choice when amitriptyline no longer works (but did), if its side effects were too severe, or if you want a sedative effect. It is well tolerated compared to the other antidepressants, but is sedating. Like desipramine, trimipramine is also used much more commonly for preventing daily headaches than for preventing migraines.

SIDE EFFECTS: Similar to amitriptyline, including constipation, sedation, a dry mouth, fatigue, and weight gain.

- **MISCELLANEOUS ANTIDEPRESSANTS (WELLBUTRIN, REMERON, EFFEXOR, SERZONE)**
  See the section in Chapter 6 for information on these antidepressants.

3. NONSTEROIDAL ANTI-INFLAMMATORIES (NSAIDS)

Commonly used to abort a headache, the NSAIDs are not as effective for preventing headaches as the antidepressants, but they do not have the antidepressants' side effects of sedation, a dry mouth, fatigue, and constipation. They do, however, often cause gastrointestinal upset (which you should report to your doctor) and potential damage to the liver and kidneys. Nevertheless, if you are under forty and suffer from arthritis, musculoskeletal problems (painful knees, back, shoulder), menstrual migraines, or the sedating effects of the antidepressants, these medications may be useful. If you are older than forty, these medications are less appropriate for daily use. The newer NSAIDs that irritate the stomach less (Vioxx, Celebrex) may be useful; their safety and effectiveness, however, have not yet been definitively established. We do not know if they will help prevent headaches; Vioxx, however, may be effective for treating a headache in progress.

Each NSAID has slightly different properties, so if one doesn't work or isn't well tolerated, your doctor may suggest trying another. If you are under age forty, it's probably worthwhile to keep searching for the right one rather than opting for a second-line medication. If you use an NSAID every day, your doctor should monitor you periodically with blood tests to be sure the medication is not causing any liver or kidney damage.

The dosing of these medications varies widely since it is important to maintain the minimum effective amount. General guidelines, however, are indicated in the list of drugs which follows. NSAIDs should always be taken with food. The NSAIDs used commonly to prevent chronic daily headache are also used to prevent migraine headaches and are discussed in more detail in Chapter 6.

- **NAPROXEN (NAPRELAN, ALEVE, NAPROSYN, ANAPROX):** 500 or 550 mg once or twice a day.
- **FLURBIPROFEN (ANSAID):** 100 to 300 mg per day.
- **KETOPROFEN (ORUDIS, ORUVAIL):** 75 to 150 mg per day.

The following NSAIDs are less commonly used for preventing tension headaches but are sometimes helpful.

- **IBUPROFEN (MOTRIN, ADVIL):** Available over the counter; 400 to 1,600 mg per day. (See Chapter 2 for a full discussion.) Ibuprofen is short-acting, rendering it less than ideal as a preventive.
- **DICLOFENAC SODIUM (VOLTAREN):** Possibly more effective than ibuprofen, 75 to 150 mg per day.
- **LODINE:** A very effective anti-inflammatory, 300 to 600 mg a day.
- **RELAFEN:** Easier on the stomach, it may be taken once or twice a day, 500 to 1,500 mg.
- **ASPIRIN:** Very inexpensive and available over the counter, two to six pills per day, 650 to 1,950 mg, enteric-coated usually recommended. (See Chapter 2 for a full discussion.)
- **COX-2 INHIBITORS:** These newer NSAIDs may cause less stomach irritation than the older kinds. Though approved by the FDA as safe, their safety and effectiveness have not yet been definitively established. Vioxx is indicated for arthritis and acute pain and may be better at treating a headache in progress than at preventing daily headaches.

If neither the antidepressants nor the nonsteroidal anti-inflammatories work to prevent your daily headaches or if you cannot tolerate their side effects, your doctor may suggest one of these second-line preventive medications.

SECOND-LINE MEDICATIONS FOR PREVENTING TENSION HEADACHES

QUICK REFERENCE GUIDE: SECOND-LINE MEDICATIONS FOR PREVENTING TENSION HEADACHES

1. NEURONTIN

A newer medication that's effective and doesn't cause stomach upset, though sedation or dizziness may occur.

2. BETA-BLOCKERS (INDERAL, CORGARD)

Occasionally useful, but cause fatigue, depression, and weight gain, and may interfere with ability to exercise.

3. MUSCLE RELAXANTS (ZANAFLEX, SKELAXIN, FLEXERIL, NORFLEX, ROBAXIN)

Only mildly effective but well tolerated. Often combined with other medications.

4. CALCIUM BLOCKERS (CALAN, ISOPTIN, VERELAN)

Occasionally effective, but often cause constipation and allergic reactions.

5. FEVERFEW

This herb can be quite effective. (See Chapter 14.)

---

1. NEURONTIN (GABAPENTIN)

A newer seizure medication (similar to Depakote), Neurontin is becoming increasingly popular for headache prevention. Neurontin is well tolerated and does not irritate the stomach or liver. However, sedation or dizziness may occur. (See Chapter 6 for a full discussion.)

2. BETA-BLOCKERS

Beta-blockers, which help prevent blood vessel dilation and may influence serotonin, are occasionally useful for tension headaches. They may, however, cause fatigue, depression, and weight gain and may interfere with your ability to exercise. The beta-blockers propranolol (Inderal) and nadolol (Corgard) are often combined with a tricyclic antidepressant or an anti-inflammatory. (See Chapter 6 for a full discussion.)

3. MUSCLE RELAXANTS

These are well-tolerated medications but usually only mildly effective. Fatigue is common and limits their usefulness, although caffeine may help counter it. Some of these medications are habit-forming, but they may be used if you have an ulcer, unlike many of the other medications. They are sometimes prescribed with an NSAID to increase pain relief, and with caffeine to counter fatigue.

- **TIZANIDINE (ZANAFLEX)**

  Approved for muscle spasticity, Zanaflex has recently been used to prevent tension or chronic daily headache. Fatigue may be a concern, although it decreases over time.

  TYPICAL DOSE: Start with one quarter or half (the tabs are double-scored) of a 4-mg tablet, at night, and increase by a quarter or half tablet in three to four days. Initially, doctors suggest using Zanaflex at night, but after four to six days, a morning dose may be added. Zanaflex may be slowly pushed up to as much as three or four in a day, in split (divided) doses.

  SIDE EFFECTS: Fatigue and drowsiness are common but decrease over time; a dry mouth is also common. Dizziness may occur.

- **METAXALONE (SKELAXIN)**

  Skelaxin has been a very reliable, safe, mild muscle relaxant; drowsiness is minimal.

  TYPICAL DOSE: One or two, two to three times per day.

  SIDE EFFECTS: While fatigue may occur, it tends to be minimal. Stomach upset, nausea, or dizziness may occur.

- **CYCLOBENZAPRINE (FLEXERIL)**

  This muscle relaxant is one of the most effective for relieving tension headaches, but it may cause severe fatigue.

  TYPICAL DOSE: Starting with 5 mg taken at night, increasing up to 10 mg twice a day if well tolerated.

  SIDE EFFECTS: Drowsiness, dizziness, lightheadedness. Less

common are confusion, a dry mouth, rapid heartbeat, and low blood pressure.

- **ORPHENADRINE (NORFLEX)**

Sometimes effective, this medication is also nonaddicting.

TYPICAL DOSE: 100 mg once or twice a day.

SIDE EFFECTS: Sedation, lightheadedness.

- **METHOCARBAMOL (ROBAXIN)**

The generic version of this medication is inexpensive, effective, and well tolerated.

TYPICAL DOSE: Starting with 250 mg at night, the dose is slowly increased to 500 or 750 mg one to three times a day.

SIDE EFFECTS: Fatigue, lightheadedness, and dizziness.

4. CALCIUM BLOCKERS (VERAPAMIL)

These medications help prevent blood vessel constriction, which may occur early in a headache, and also influence serotonin. They are occasionally effective but often cause constipation and allergic reactions. Verapamil (Calan, Isoptin, Verelan) is the most effective calcium blocker. (See Chapter 6 for a full discussion.)

If the first- and second-line therapies don't help, there are a few more possible avenues to take.

5. FEVERFEW

Feverfew is a relatively safe herb that may help prevent migraine and daily headaches. There are a number of preparations available. (See Chapters 6 and 14 for details.)

THIRD-LINE MEDICATIONS FOR PREVENTING TENSION HEADACHES

QUICK REFERENCE GUIDE: THIRD-LINE MEDICATIONS FOR PREVENTING TENSION HEADACHES

1. COMBINING TWO PREVENTIVES

Increases risk of side effects but could enhance effectiveness.

2. MAO Inhibitors (Phenelzine [Nardil])

Powerful and sometimes the only thing that works, but strict dietary restrictions are necessary, and weight gain and insomnia are common.

3. Intravenous DHE

Sometimes useful, but requires doctor visits.

4. Tranquilizers (Klonopin, Librium, Valium, phenobarbital)

Occasionally does the trick better than anything else, but can be habit-forming.

5. Amphetamines (Ritalin, Dexedrine)

A last resort; chemical dependency, insomnia, and anxiety are potential problems.

6. Daily Long-Acting Narcotics (Dolophine, Oxycontin, Kadian, MS Contin)

Provides excellent relief but sedation and constipation are common. May be habit-forming.

1. Taking Two Preventive Medications

If you are extremely frustrated with moderate or severe headaches and want quick results, or if you suddenly get severe headaches (usually a combination of daily tension headaches and migraines) that you can't deal with, your doctor may suggest pushing the preventive strategy ahead at a faster pace by suggesting that you try two preventive medications. Sometimes when one preventive medication doesn't work, two will. The various preventive medications possess different mechanisms of action.

Common combinations include a tricyclic antidepressant with an NSAID or a beta-blocker; an NSAID with a beta-blocker or a calcium blocker; amitriptyline with propranolol; sometimes valproate (Depakote) with an antidepressant, beta-blocker, or calcium blocker. One or two preventive medications may also be prescribed at the same time as repetitive IV DHE (description follows).

Although the risk of side effects increases with two medications, this treatment is justified if your headaches severely compromise your quality of life.

2. MAO INHIBITORS (PHENELZINE)

Phenelzine (Nardil) is a powerful medication for migraines and daily headaches (and for depression and anxiety). Sometimes it is the only thing that works. Its use is limited, however, because of strict dietary restrictions (see "Third-Line Medications for Preventing Migraines" in Chapter 6). Some people also object to the common side effects of weight gain and insomnia.

3. REPETITIVE INTRAVENOUS (IV) DHE

Although IV DHE is most effective for migraines, it is sometimes useful for daily headaches as well. If you are dependent on analgesics, your doctor may prescribe DHE to help you withdraw from them. It's a safe medication but expensive. (See Chapter 6 for a full discussion.)

4. TRANQUILIZERS

Although only occasionally effective for daily headaches, a tranquilizer is just the right medication for some people. These drugs can, however, be habit-forming so doctors will usually minimize doses and carefully monitor you if you go on one of them.

- **CLONAZEPAM (KLONOPIN)**
  Useful for insomnia and anxiety.
- **CHLORDIAZEPOXIDE (LIBRIUM)**
  Relatively mild and well tolerated.
- **DIAZEPAM (VALIUM)**
  Can be useful but habit-forming.
- **PHENOBARBITAL**
  May help with anxiety as well as preventing headaches.

5. AMPHETAMINES

These are last-resort medications that are somewhat effective and generally well tolerated, but they can lead to chemical dependency. Insomnia and anxiety are also potential problems. Typical amphetamines used for preventing tension headaches are methylphenidate (Ritalin) or dextroamphetamine (Dexedrine). See Chapter 6 for details.

6. DAILY LONG-ACTING NARCOTIC OPIOIDS

The longer-acting opioids, such as methadone (Dolophine), Oxycontin, and Kadian or MS Contin have been used for chronic cancer pain. For those with constant, chronic moderate, or severe pain, these medications sometimes provide excellent relief. The advantage of longer-acting opioids is that they help for eight to twelve hours, as opposed to the shorter-acting medications (such as Tylenol with codeine, Vicodin, and Darvocet). These are actually *less* addictive than the short-acting opioids. (See Chapter 6 for details. Also see Chapter 5 for a discussion of addiction versus dependence.)

CASE STUDIES

Here are several case studies, showing how all this information on tension headaches might be applied.

PHYLLIS

INITIAL VISIT: Phyllis is a twenty-seven-year-old woman who is home with a young child. She reports that she first began getting chronic daily headaches at sixteen, but they stopped for a few years, from age twenty-two through twenty-four. They have since returned and are now severe. Occasionally Phyllis gets a migraine, but her primary problem is the daily headache. It hurts all over her head as "an aching pressure" and is present all the time, "twenty-four hours a day." She says that over-the-counter medications are of no use. Relaxation techniques do help, but she does not want to do the deep breathing and imaging. The headaches are not increased by any triggers that Phyllis can identify. She says, "Whether I am under no stress or great stress, the headache is there all the time, day after day, and is just the same. It hurts a lot." Chiropractic and massage therapy helped for one or two days, but only minimally. Allergy testing, dental (TMJ) testing, and eye tests were all normal.

Phyllis's doctor prescribes 10 mg of amitriptyline (Elavil) as a preventive medication to be taken at night.

WEEK 6: Phyllis cannot tolerate Elavil because she gained weight and was very tired, even on this low dose. Her doctor prescribes fluoxetine (Prozac), 20 mg each morning, as Prozac usually causes very little sedation or dryness in the mouth.

WEEK 10: Phyllis suffers no side effects from the Prozac, but the medication works only moderately well; she says the pain is "fifty percent" better and wants more relief. Her dose of Prozac is raised to 40 mg a day.

WEEK 13: Phyllis calls her doctor to say she's still getting a headache every day and that the 40 mg of Prozac is making her feel tired and "spacy." The doctor lowers the dose again to 20 mg and prescribes the anti-inflammatory naproxen (anti-inflammatories as preventive medications are prescribed much more in Phyllis's relatively young age range than for older patients).

WEEK 16: Phyllis reports that she is getting no additional relief and the doctor takes her off the naproxen, which carries the risk of gastrointestinal, kidney, and liver side effects. He adds nortriptyline (Pamelor), 10 mg, at night. Phyllis gains some weight, but the headaches are 75 percent improved, and she wishes to stay on Prozac plus Pamelor.

THE FUTURE: If Phyllis is willing, she can try other preventive medications, such as other antidepressants or valproate (Depakote), but she prefers to stick with her current regimen for now. Beta-blockers, such as propranolol, are also possibilities. Gabapentin (Neurontin) is also a good possibility.

HEATHER

INITIAL VISIT: Heather is a thirty-three-year-old stockbroker with a history of severe daily tension headache and one migraine monthly. She's had the daily headaches since age sixteen, but they didn't become severe until two years ago. Her job is very stressful, as is her marriage. When Heather saw a physician last year, she was taking sixteen aspirin plus over-the-counter caffeine tablets and six ibuprofen tablets a day. Her blood tests revealed that her liver was irritated and she was having severe stomach pains due to the stress and medicine.

Heather's physician took her off the aspirin and ibuprofen and prescribed Esgic (a butalbital compound with acetaminophen and caffeine), but Heather is now consuming ten Esgic tablets a day.

She is experiencing some degree of analgesic rebound headache, in which her medication is actually creating more pain for her the next day. This is a common problem and usually occurs when someone takes more than four or five pain relievers (though can range from as little as two to as many as eight) a day.

Heather tapers off the painkillers and gets four injections of intravenous DHE, which is commonly used to help people withdraw from analgesics and to relieve the headaches for a period of time. The key with Heather is to avoid painkillers and to find an effective daily preventive medication.

The physician prescribes nortriptyline (Pamelor), a tricyclic antidepressant that is somewhat milder than amitriptyline (Elavil). They hope that the medication will prevent both the daily tension headache as well as the monthly migraine. Heather also receives a prescription for sumatriptan (Imitrex) tablets for the migraines, but the plan is simply to use preventive medications for her daily pain.

WEEK 4: Heather has successfully withdrawn from the analgesics with the DHE breaking the cycle of rebound headaches. The nortriptyline has helped prevent headaches, but her blood tests continue to show some liver irritation, which may have been caused by the nortriptyline. Her daily preventive medication is changed to paroxetine (Paxil), 10 mg each morning.

WEEK 6: The Paxil is not helping, so the dose is raised to 20 mg each morning. The liver tests have returned to normal. Heather is not allowed to consume any daily painkillers.

WEEK 7: The tension headaches are only about 25 percent improved with the Paxil, so Heather switches back to nortriptyline and the dose is slowly increased to the point at which the headaches are 70 percent improved in severity. Her liver tests remain normal. The monthly migraines are gone.

Analgesic rebound headaches can be relatively easily controlled once someone is no longer taking pain medications. The key is to find a preventive medication that will work. In rare situations, in which all of the prevention approaches have failed, daily pain medications may be used in controlled amounts; twelve or fourteen tablets of an analgesic per day is unacceptable. Imitrex works well for Heather's migraines.

THE FUTURE: If the nortriptyline stops working or produces unacceptable side effects in the future, there are many other options, including other antidepressants; beta-blockers, such as propranolol (Inderal); verapamil (Isoptin); and valproate (Depakote). Depakote may be the best option; Neurontin is also a possibility. For her migraines, Heather may consider Imitrex injections if the tablets are no longer effective.

LOUIS

INITIAL VISIT: Louis, a forty-two-year-old accountant, has had daily headaches for almost two decades. They hurt in a "hatband" fashion around his head and increase in severity as the day goes on. He reports that they are worse with stress and weather changes, if he drinks red wine, or if he eats food that contains MSG. The headaches wax and wane, and occasionally Louis goes four or five days without one.

For four years, Louis used two Excedrin Extra-Strength tablets a day to control his pain. Relaxation techniques and exercise have not helped. Massage helps for one day, but then the pain returns. Louis has sought relief, but to no avail, from chiropractors, allergists, dentists, sinus doctors, and eye doctors.

He began needing more and more Excedrin, to the point of taking eight a day. His stomach began to hurt (due to the aspirin in the Excedrin), and his headaches were getting worse. All the Excedrin was evidently giving Louis rebound headaches. His doctor takes him off Excedrin and places him on an antidepressant as preventive medication, protriptyline (Vivactil). The doctor chooses Vivactil over amitriptyline because it is not sedating and never causes weight gain; he chooses it over fluoxetine (Prozac), Paxil, or Zoloft because it is more effective. Vivactil can keep people up at night, but Louis does not have insomnia.

WEEK 8: On Vivactil, the headaches decrease to the point where Louis has almost no pain, but he has side effects from the medication, particularly constipation, a dry mouth, and insomnia. His doctor prescribes Depakote instead. While Prozac is still a possibility, Louis and his doctor decide not to continue with an antidepressant for now because of Louis's problems with Vivactil's side effects.

WEEK 12: Although Louis hasn't called the office between visits, he now reports that the Depakote helped only a bit. On his own, he went back to taking aspirin and caffeine in the form of Anacin. Once again he crept up to taking eight a day, and once more the headaches increased because of the analgesic rebound situation. A stressful divorce further increased the headaches, and Louis began mixing ibuprofen with the aspirin and caffeine. He developed an ulcer and was hospitalized. At this point, his doctor takes him off the analgesics and gives him five injections of IV DHE, which greatly helps the headaches. The doctor prescribes nortriptyline (Pamelor), a mild antidepressant, 25 mg at night, as a preventive medication. This dose is low. As nortriptyline may cause constipation (and a dry mouth), Louis's doctor informs him about how to minimize this problem through a proper diet and laxatives if necessary.

WEEK 20: Louis reports that he does get a mild dry mouth from the medication, but that the preventive medication (the antidepressant with no analgesics) is quite successful in that he is now getting relatively few headaches. He estimates that the pain is 80 percent better. Because this improvement is within the range of success expected with preventive medications, Louis agrees to continue on the nortriptyline. Although weight gain with nortriptyline can be a major problem, it is not in Louis's case.

THE FUTURE: If the current dose of nortriptyline begins

to lose its effectiveness, the doctor may increase the dose. Or he and Louis may want to consider Neurontin. Alternative antidepressants, such as Prozac, Zoloft, Paxil, Effexor, or Serzone, may also help.

JOSEPH

INITIAL VISIT: Joseph is a sixty-eight-year-old executive with a history of chronic daily headache, moderate in intensity, and frequent, sharp pains in the back of his head, on the right side only, lasting up to one minute. The sharp pains are diagnosed as occipital neuralgia (to read more about this condition, see Chapter 13). Joseph has had headaches since he was twenty-six, but they have gotten worse in the past several years. Stress, certain foods, and golf exacerbate them. His mother and two of his three children have a history of headaches. Joseph has had ulcers and has high blood pressure. He reports that over-the-counter medications have ceased working for him and that he has tried several prescription acetaminophen-based analgesics, but none of them has been effective.

Joseph's doctor instructs him in the nonmedication aspects of headaches, but relaxation techniques are generally ineffective for his age range. The doctor prescribes propranolol (Inderal), a high blood pressure medication, as a preventive. Because of Joseph's advanced age, the doctor keeps the dose low to minimize side effects. Although an antidepressant may be more effective, Joseph's doctor chooses propranolol to lessen his medication over the long term and because it should stabilize his blood pressure as well.

For an abortive medication, Joseph receives a prescription for butalbital with acetaminophen (Phrenilin) and instructions to take no more than two per day. Any more could lead to rebound headaches. To alleviate the sharp pains in the back of his head, Joseph gets an injection of bupivacaine (Marcaine) in that area. This procedure is easy and safe and takes just minutes in the doctor's office yet it can provide weeks or even months of relief.

WEEK 4: Joseph reports that his headaches are about 20 percent better on the Inderal. His blood pressure is under control. The novocaine injection provided three weeks of relief for the pains in the back of the head, but they have started to return. The doctor increases the Inderal dose.

WEEK 6: Joseph calls to say the increased dose does not help and leaves him tired. The doctor reduces the Inderal dose. To supplement Joseph's preventive medication, the doctor prescribes nortriptyline (10 mg of Pamelor, quickly raised to 25 mg), a mild antidepressant, to take at night because it helps sleeping. The Phrenilin is continued as an abortive, to be taken when needed.

WEEK 12: Joseph calls to say his headaches are 70 percent better, but he is very tired and constipated. These side effects are from the Pamelor, so the doctor lowers the dose back to 10 mg. Joseph also reports that the Phrenilin no longer relieves the headache once it starts, so he and his doctor agree that he should discontinue the medication and stick to daily preventives. Because of his ulcer problems, Joseph can't use aspirin or anti-inflammatories as abortives, and many of the other choices are too strong and cause too many side effects. The aspirin-NSAID medications are prescribed infrequently for older people because of the increased risk of side effects with advancing age. Joseph and his doctor discuss the possibility of a very small amount of daily narcotic analgesic, such as hydrocodone, but they consider it a last resort. For now, Joseph will use the daily preventives and not chase after the pain every four hours.

WEEK 16: Joseph reports that his headaches are about 40 percent better than they were before his first visit. The low 10-mg dose of Pamelor helps somewhat and does not make him tired. He remains on the Inderal for the blood pressure and headaches.

THE FUTURE: Other considerations, if needed, may be one of the SSRI (selective serotonin reuptake inhibitor) antidepressants, such as Prozac, Zoloft, or Paxil, all of which are used for headaches. These medications have been very useful because they generally do not cause sedation, weight gain, or constipation. However, they do have some side effects, such as anxiety, nausea, decreased libido or sexual performance, and insomnia. In addition, other blood pressure medications may help Joseph, such as different beta-blockers (Corgard, Lopressor, Tenormin) or calcium blockers (Isoptin, Calan). Depakote or Neurontin are also good possibilities. If possible, daily painkillers will be avoided. Zanaflex, a muscle relaxant, is also a possibility.

10

· · · · · · · ·

UNDERSTANDING AND TREATING CLUSTER HEADACHES

CLUSTER HEADACHES, though uncommon, are one of the most painful experiences known to humankind. Approximately one out of 250 men, and one out of 800 women, will live with this misery. If you are one of the unfortunate few who get them, you may suffer terribly, as they can be excruciating and debilitating. The pain may last anywhere from fifteen minutes to three hours, occasionally longer. Usually, the pain sears through or around one eye, or locates itself in the temple. These headaches are called cluster headaches because they occur in waves, a series of headaches lasting several weeks to several months, once or twice a year, most commonly in the spring and fall. Occasionally, the intervals between attacks are much longer.

WHAT ARE CLUSTER HEADACHES?

Three to four times more common among men than women, cluster headaches cause extreme and sudden pain without any warning or aura. Although experts assume that serotonin imbalances cause clusters, they also think that a malfunctioning of the body's biological clock, the hypothalamus, may also be involved because of the cyclic nature of these headaches. This malfunctioning might be due to subtle structural brain differences in people who get cluster headaches. Using the latest imaging technology to peer into the brain, researchers have reported recently that the density of brain matter in people who get cluster headaches is significantly different from that of people who don't get the headaches. This area of the brain affected is what controls the body's biological clock, which could be why cluster headaches strike with such regularity, at certain times of day or night. Cluster headaches are probably one of the vascular headaches, as are migraines, partly caused by constricting and dilating blood vessels — probably of the carotid artery close to the eye — but surrounding nerves are also involved. Since smokers have a higher rate of cluster headaches, subtle changes in the bloodstream that may occur in smokers probably also play a role.

Usually cluster headaches start between ages twenty and forty-five. If you first got cluster headaches early in life, you may outgrow them by your fifties; people who start getting cluster headaches later in life have a greater chance of having chronic cluster headaches.

A cluster headache often begins with a sense of fullness in one ear and then progresses to a stab of pain near the eye, forehead, or cheek, sometimes even as low as the jaw. Within minutes, the pain can become excruciating. For most people, the pain remains on the same side, though occasionally it may switch to the other, either during the same cluster cycle or in the next cycle. Your eye will probably tear and your nose will run on the same side as the pain.

On average, attacks last forty-five minutes, starting at the same time of day, usually during the night. Typically, they build in intensity over days or weeks. The series of headaches most commonly consists of one or two headaches a day for three to eight weeks (sometimes for as long as five months), once or twice a year. These clusters are called "intermittent" or "episodic." About one in ten sufferers has "chronic" cluster headaches, with less than a six-month break between cycles.

The pain may be extremely intense, "like an eye is being pulled out." Many people writhe in agony, rock, or bang their heads against the wall. Some sufferers say that the pain is worse than it would be if a limb were cut off in an accident. In contrast to migraine sufferers, who seek a dark, quiet room and lie still, people who are suffering from cluster headaches tend to pace about.

Cluster headaches are often misdiagnosed as a sinus or allergy problem because of the runny or stuffed nose and teary eye. You can probably identify your headaches as clusters if they follow this pattern:

- Onset between ages twenty and forty-five
- Most common among men (three to four times more than in women)
- Occur same time of year, with no headache between the cluster cycles
- Attacks usually occur at night
- During a cycle, alcohol is the most common trigger
- Severe, excruciating pain on one side, usually around the eye
- Eye tearing (lacrimation) and red on the side of the pain
- Small pupil (miosis of the pupil)
- Drooping eyelid
- Stuffed or runny nostril on the side of the pain
- Sweaty face or forehead (on the side of the pain)

NONDRUG STRATEGIES TO TREAT CLUSTER HEADACHES

Unfortunately, very little except medication really helps cluster headaches. The pain is too severe for relaxation methods, although a few simple deep-breathing exercises can help you cope with the dread and anticipation of another cluster. People in the midst of a series are often extremely anxious, fearing a night of intense, excruciating pain.

Applying ice to the painful area may help, although some people prefer heat. A hot shower massager with moderate pressure on the scalp may also ease some pain.

Once a cluster series has started, sensitivity to alcohol is much greater and often can trigger an attack. The other typical headache foods are less important, although you should avoid especially MSG, and to some extent, aged cheeses, aged meats, and chocolate during a cluster series. Occasionally, certain triggers, such as the letdown after stress, excessive cold or heat, or bright light may bring on a cluster. By and large, however, you can't control the time when a cluster will strike, except perhaps with medication.

TREATING CLUSTER HEADACHES WITH MEDICATION

If you get either intermittent or chronic cluster headaches, you will probably cope best if you have medication both to treat and to prevent an attack. Since the pain is very sudden, intense, and relatively brief, lasting less than an hour, the abortive medication must act quickly. Taking medication by mouth usually isn't fast enough. An oral pain reliever is more useful if your attacks typically last more than an hour. Antinausea medication is sometimes used, not only to combat nausea but for its sedative effect as well.

QUICK REFERENCE GUIDE:
TREATING CLUSTER HEADACHES

FIRST-LINE MEDICATIONS

1. SUMATRIPTAN (IMITREX) INJECTION OR NASAL SPRAY
Injections are fast and highly effective.

2. OXYGEN
Easy and inexpensive, inhalations work for 60 percent of cases.

3. ERGOTAMINE TARTRATE
Suppositories most effective, but medication often triggers side effects, especially anxiety and nausea.

4. DHE INJECTIONS
Effective but doesn't come in prepackaged auto-injectors.

SECOND-LINE MEDICATIONS

1. PAIN RELIEVERS — ANTI-INFLAMMATORIES AND NARCOTICS
Trial and error at this point; narcotics can be addicting.

---

2. LIDOCAINE NASAL SPRAY
Useful in combination with other medications
3. KETOROLAC (TORADOL) INJECTIONS
Can be effective and fast; a nonsedating, nonaddictive anti-inflammatory.
4. ANTINAUSEA MEDICATIONS
In addition to easing nausea, can promote sedation.

FIRST-LINE MEDICATIONS FOR ABORTING CLUSTER HEADACHES

When you first go to a doctor about cluster headaches, chances are that he will recommend one of these treatments to relieve the pain after the headache has started.

1. SUMATRIPTAN (IMITREX) INJECTION OR NASAL SPRAY
Imitrex is even more effective for cluster headaches than for migraine headaches. After an injection, the pain may stop in as little as three to five minutes. The nasal spray is milder and may take twenty to thirty minutes to work. The nasal spray should be used on the opposite side of the headache (since your nose will probably be stuffed up on the same side).

The tablets are usually too slow to act; however, if you get prolonged cluster headaches (longer than one hour), you may prefer them. Long-term side effects of daily triptans (such as Imitrex) are not yet known. The other triptans (Amerge, Maxalt, Zomig, Relpax) take longer to work than the Imitrex injections and nasal spray, but may be helpful for prolonged cluster headaches. (See Chapter 5 for more details.)

2. OXYGEN
This treatment involves inhaling oxygen from a tank. It is very effective in 60 percent of cases, and renting a tank and mask is relatively easy and moderately inexpensive.

To use the oxygen tank, sit, leaning slightly forward. Inhale 100 percent oxygen (8 liters per minute) with the mask, for fifteen to twenty minutes, longer if needed, but no more than one hour a day, assuming you have no pulmonary problems. Oxygen may be used at the same time as Imitrex or ergotamine.

3. ERGOTAMINE TARTRATE

A moderately effective blood vessel constrictor, ergotamine tartrate has many side effects, especially severe anxiety and nausea. Although this medication presents the risk of rebound headaches when used with migraines, they do not occur with cluster headaches.

Unlike sumatriptan and DHE, in which the most effective form is an injection, ergotamine tartrate can be effective in pill form, though suppositories are most effective. After age forty, this medication must be used with caution because of the risk for heart complications.

(For details about specific medications in this group, see Chapter 5.)

4. DIHYDROERGOTAMINE (DHE)

Similar to sumatriptan, DHE is somewhat less effective but lasts longer and has been on the market for years. Unlike sumatriptan, it is not available in premeasured auto-injectors or in pill form, though it is available in a nasal spray (Migranal Nasal Spray). Injections, however, are the most effective form.

If you have any kind of heart disease, DHE must be used with caution. (For more details, see Chapter 5.)

SECOND-LINE MEDICATIONS FOR
ABORTING CLUSTER HEADACHES

When the first-line medications don't work, there are other options.

1. PAIN RELIEVERS

At this stage of headache management, the doctor may suggest anything ranging from over-the-counter Excedrin Extra-Strength and Excedrin Migraine to naproxen (Aleve, Anaprox DS), butal-bital compounds (Fiorinal or Esgic), or perhaps narcotics, all of which we discuss in detail in Chapter 5. These may be combined with oxygen, Imitrex, or ergotamines. Because addiction is always a potential problem with narcotics, you should resort to them only when the milder options don't work. (See Chapter 5 for a discussion of addiction versus dependence.)

2. Lidocaine Nasal Spray

Though rarely useful by itself for treating clusters, lidocaine spray may be recommended in combination with other methods. It is mildly effective but safe, easy to use, and has minimal side effects. Lidocaine may be useful while waiting for the abortives to work.

TYPICAL DOSE: The pharmacist will put 4 percent lidocaine (from a bottle) into a plastic nasal spray container. Lie down, with your head extended back, and turn your head toward the side of the pain. Spray two or three times but no more than eight in twenty-four hours. If a spray bottle is unavailable, 1 ml of 4 percent lidocaine can be dropped with an eye dropper into the nostril near the pain.

SIDE EFFECTS: Sometimes temporary numbness in the throat. Nervousness and rapid heartbeat occur rarely.

3. Ketorolac (Toradol) Injections

Ketorolac is an effective and fast-acting anti-inflammatory when injected. It is nonsedating and nonaddictive and is available in pill form but must be injected for most effective relief. Prefilled syringes are available, as well as individual vials.

TYPICAL DOSE: 60 mg in a prefilled syringe or a vial, repeated half an hour or an hour later if needed, with 30 mg or 60 mg. No more than three injections per week.

SIDE EFFECTS: Use should be monitored and limited during a series of cluster headaches, to avoid kidney and liver complications. Because ketorolac is an anti-inflammatory, it may cause stomach pain.

(See Chapter 5 for more details.)

4. ANTINAUSEA MEDICATION

These medications can help any nausea that occurs, as well as promote sedation, which is sometimes desired to tolerate the cluster.

- **PROMETHAZINE (PHENERGAN)**
  Promethazine is sedating but has few other side effects. Available in pill or suppository form, promethazine also helps enhance the effectiveness of pain relievers.
- **PROCHLORPERAZINE (COMPAZINE) AND CHLORPROMAZINE (THORAZINE)**
  These are stronger antinausea medications that are useful to promote sedation when you want to avoid going to the emergency room for your pain.
  (See Chapter 5 for more details.)

PREVENTING CLUSTER HEADACHES

When abortive medications don't relieve your cluster headaches and your headaches occur daily for longer than fifteen minutes, most doctors will recommend a preventive. You may choose to take daily preventive medication as soon as a series begins because the headaches are extremely severe and difficult to relieve when in progress. But to take preventive medications, you must be willing to take daily medicine for the length of the cluster series and endure the possible side effects. If you get chronic, rather than intermittent, cluster headaches, you'll probably do best if you take daily medication year-round or at least while the headaches are severe.

Once you are certain that a cluster cycle has begun, your doctor may recommend that you start taking cortisone, the fastest-acting of the first-line preventive medications, along with another medication in this group, either lithium or verapamil. The theory is that by the time the cortisone is withdrawn (it shouldn't be taken for too long), the second preventive will have become effective.

When your cluster series ends, the medication can be stopped a week or two after the last headache and not started up again until the first signs of another series. After discovering what's effective and tolerable for you, your doctor will probably recommend that you institute the same regimen whenever you think a cluster series is beginning, which often occurs at the same time of the year.

QUICK REFERENCE GUIDE:

PREVENTING CLUSTER HEADACHES

FIRST-LINE MEDICATIONS

1. CORTISONE

Very effective but side effects are common: nervousness, moodiness, sleep problems, fatigue, stomach pain.

2. VERAPAMIL

Well-tolerated calcium blocker but takes days to weeks to become fully effective. Can aggravate daily headaches (tension type).

3. LITHIUM

Useful, especially when taken with one of the above, but numerous possible side effects.

SECOND-LINE MEDICATIONS

1. METHYSERGIDE (SANSERT)

Sometimes effective but has many side effects.

2. VALPROATE (DEPAKOTE)

Sometimes very useful, but may often cause lethargy and gastrointestinal problems.

3. ERGOTAMINES (CAFERGOT, BELLERGAL-S)

Not for anyone over forty-five or with high blood pressure, heart disease, or vascular problems.

4. ERGONOVINE (ERGOTRATE)

Well tolerated but not as effective as above medications.

5. DAILY TRIPTANS

Occasionally effective.

6. INDOMETHACIN (INDOCIN)

May be just the right thing for some people, but sometimes triggers stomach pain.

---

7. STEROID BLOCKADE
Can relieve pain for weeks if other drugs fail; injection is given under the skin at the back of the head.

THIRD-LINE MEDICATIONS

1. IV DHE
Can quickly reduce frequency of headaches while you wait for another preventive medication to kick in.

2. COCAINE SOLUTION
When nothing else works, during peak problem times.

FIRST-LINE MEDICATIONS FOR
PREVENTING CLUSTER HEADACHES

As with migraines, the effects of these medications are cumulative, so if one medication is not completely effective, the doctor may recommend a combination of verapamil, lithium, and cortisone. Lithium with verapamil is a common combination for clusters, with or without using cortisone for brief periods.

1. CORTISONE

Prednisone, dexamethasone (Decadron), triamcinolone (Aristocort), or an injectable form (Depo-Medrol).

Cortisone is very effective and used primarily for episodic clusters. Side effects are likely, as your physician and medication package insert will explain. Cluster headache sufferers usually take cortisone for just one or two weeks during the peak of the series.

TYPICAL DOSE: Should be as small as possible and taken with food. Prednisone, 20 mg (or Decadron, 4 mg) once a day for three days, then 10 mg of prednisone (half a pill) per day for six to ten days. Injectable forms provide quick relief for up to a week, usually not longer. Additional cortisone may be used later in the cycle if the clusters increase.

SIDE EFFECTS: Nervousness, moodiness, and sleep problems; when used for brief periods, side effects are usually minimal.

Sometimes fluid retention, fatigue, gastrointestinal upset, and stomach pain.

2. VERAPAMIL (CALAN, ISOPTIN, VERELAN, COVERA-HS)

Verapamil is a well-tolerated calcium blocker with minimal side effects, though it may aggravate or cause chronic daily headaches. It is effective for episodic and chronic clusters, but needs to be taken for at least several days and sometimes several weeks to become fully effective.

TYPICAL DOSE: 240 mg slow-release or long-acting pill once or twice a day. At the start of a headache, verapamil is often prescribed with cortisone and then still taken after cortisone is discontinued.

SIDE EFFECTS: Constipation, allergic reactions (rashes), dizziness, insomnia, anxiety, and occasionally fatigue.

3. LITHIUM

Lithium is usually well tolerated when taken in low doses. It can be very helpful for chronic clusters and, to a lesser degree, episodic clusters. It is commonly combined with verapamil or cortisone.

TYPICAL DOSE: 300 to 900 mg a day, occasionally higher.

SIDE EFFECTS: Drowsiness, mood swings, nausea, vomiting, thirst, tremor, diarrhea. Low doses and good monitoring usually prevent serious problems that can occur otherwise.

SECOND-LINE MEDICATIONS FOR PREVENTING CLUSTER HEADACHES

When first-line medications do not reliably prevent cluster headaches, a physician may progress to one of these medications, which we describe in more detail earlier in the book.

1. METHYSERGIDE (SANSERT)

Somewhat effective for episodic clusters but not usually for chronic clusters, Sansert can be useful but has many potential side effects, such as nausea, leg cramps, and dizziness. It is not, however, generally recommended for people with active peptic ulcers, peripheral vascular disease, cardiac valve problems, coronary artery disease, high blood pressure, kidney or liver problems, or for those who are pregnant or over forty-five. (See Chapter 6 for a full discussion.)

2. VALPROATE (DEPAKOTE)

A seizure medication that is often used for cluster, migraine, and tension headaches, valproate is sometimes very useful but it may cause lethargy, gastrointestinal upset, mood swings, weight gain, and hair loss.

It is fairly well tolerated, but nausea, gastritis (stomach pain or burning), sedation, emotional upset (depression or mood swings), hair loss, rashes, and dose-related tremors may occur. If taken for months, weight gain is common but is usually limited. Liver functions and blood counts need to be monitored closely in the first several months, but for episodic clusters, the entire duration of use is only one or two months, and one blood test is usually adequate. (See Chapter 6 for a full discussion.)

3. ERGOTAMINES (CAFERGOT, BELLERGAL-S, ERGOMAR, ERGONOVINE)

While headache doctors do not usually prescribe daily ergotamines (blood vessel constrictors), because of the risk of long-term effects and rebound headaches (common in migraine patients), the risk is much smaller in cluster sufferers who typically use the medication for a briefer period, only four to eight weeks, and stop after an episode is over.

Great caution must be taken by people who are older than around age forty. Ergotamines are not usually recommended for anyone with high blood pressure, heart disease, or vascular disease in the legs.

TYPICAL DOSE: Most effective when taken within several hours of the expected cluster attack. If a headache typically occurs at eleven P.M., then optimal timing of the drug is nine or ten P.M. The usual dose is 1 or 2 mg (up to 4 mg) per day.

- **CAFERGOT** pills or suppositories may be used as the source of ergotamine, but the 100 mg of caffeine increases side effects.
- **BELLERGAL-S** is comprised of ergotamine, phenobarbital (a sedative), and belladonna. The sedating effect of phenobarbital is occasionally helpful for the cluster patient, but the relatively low dose of ergotamine (0.6 mg) is usually insufficient to prevent an attack.

SIDE EFFECTS: Nausea and nervousness, fatigue, muscle aches, tingling, numbing in the hands or feet, chest pain. (See Chapter 5 for more details.)

4. ERGONOVINE (ERGOTRATE)

A well-tolerated medication, ergonovine is generally not as effective as methysergide but it poses fewer side effects.

TYPICAL DOSE: 0.2 mg, two to four times a day.

SIDE EFFECTS: Mild gastrointestinal upset, anxiety.

5. DAILY TRIPTANS

Occasionally, the long-acting daily triptan, Amerge, may be effective (taken once or twice per day) in preventing episodic cluster headache. Occasionally, sumatriptan (Imitrex) is used in this way. Triptans are not approved for this use, and the long-term safety of daily use has not been firmly established. If you are using tablets of Imitrex, then you might try injections as needed for an acute cluster headache. If your doctor has recommended that you take one or two tablets per day of Imitrex preventively, Imitrex Nasal Spray may be used on an "as-needed" basis.

Generally, daily triptans are only occasionally successful in preventing cluster headaches. However, if most of the first-line and second-line approaches have not been successful, you might need to try some last-resort efforts. To use a triptan preventively, time the triptan for one hour or so prior to the expected onset of a cluster headache. Since most people experience more of the clusters at night, try to time the triptan in the evening before you would usually experience the pain. So far, side effects haven't been a problem with this approach, because it is usually used for relatively short periods of time.

6. INDOMETHACIN (INDOCIN)

Indomethacin is an anti-inflammatory that is unique because it may be effective for certain types of headache when other similar medications are not. Indomethacin may cause stomach pain or upset, but it is usually relatively well tolerated. It is very useful in the variation of cluster headache called chronic paroxysmal hemicrania (see Chapter 13). Unlike some of the preventive medications, it is apparent within days whether Indomethacin will be effective.

TYPICAL DOSE: From 75 mg to 225 mg per day, taken with food.

7. STEROID BLOCKADE OF THE OCCIPITAL NERVE (CORTISONE)

When other drugs cannot control a headache, sufferers can use this therapy at the peak of the series. By placing cortisone (such as Depo-Medrol or betamethasone) in the region of the greater occipital nerve, a cluster can be relieved somewhat for up to weeks at a time. These medications are well tolerated, with few side effects.

TYPICAL DOSE: 60 to 80 mg of Depo-Medrol per injection. An injection may be repeated once, if necessary, but two injections per cluster series is generally the maximum.

SIDE EFFECTS: Infection, discoloration, or dimpling of skin, though rare, may occur. Stomach pain, anxiety, or insomnia may also occur.

For a full discussion on treating occipital neuralgia, see Chapter 13.

THIRD-LINE MEDICATIONS FOR
PREVENTING EPISODIC CLUSTER HEADACHES

If none of these strategies works for you, your doctor may recommend either intravenous DHE, administered repetitively, or a cocaine solution to be used nasally during the day to prevent the clusters.

1. Intravenous Dihydroergotamine (IV DHE)

Intravenous DHE can quickly cut down on the number of cluster headaches you get and can control clusters while you wait for a preventive medication (such as verapamil or lithium) to take effect. Its pain-relieving effects may last for weeks.

(See Chapter 6 for a full discussion of IV DHE.)

2. Cocaine Solution (A last-resort, end-of-the-line therapy)

If your episodic cluster series lasts several months and all other preventive measures have failed, cocaine may help you. It is particularly useful during a peak season of chronic clusters. The treatment involves using a 10 percent solution during the day to reduce the number and severity of the clusters. This dose rarely produces any euphoric or cognitive effects.

Addiction risk may be a problem (and its use generally would not be recommended if you have any addiction history), but the low concentration, high cost, and difficulty in obtaining the solution makes cocaine a last-resort therapy.

TYPICAL DOSE: One or two drops in each nostril one to four times a day. If the clusters are severe and out of control, your doctor may suggest beginning with two drops four times a day, quickly cutting the dose down to as little as is effective. Usually limited to two grams of cocaine in two months.

SIDE EFFECTS: Occasional nervousness or insomnia; euphoric effects of cocaine may occur but not commonly. If euphoria is experienced, the percentage of cocaine should be cut down to 4 percent or stopped completely. The patient must understand the addiction potential.

ADDITIONAL TREATMENTS FOR EPISODIC CLUSTER HEADACHES

Occasionally, other medications may help cluster headaches, including phenelzine, cyproheptadine, nifedipine, beta-blockers, antidepressants, long-acting daily opiods, or methylphenidate (Ritalin).

- **PHENELZINE (NARDIL),** an MAO inhibitor, is a powerful anti-migraine medication that is occasionally useful for cluster headaches. (See Chapter 6 for more details.)

- **CYPROHEPTADINE (PERIACTIN)** is occasionally helpful for clusters, but its effect is usually very mild. Side effects, such as fatigue and weight gain, are often problems. Best when used with other therapies for clusters.

- **NIFEDIPINE (PROCARDIA),** a well-tolerated calcium blocker, is as effective as verapamil for many cluster patients. However, if verapamil does not work, the nifedipine usually is ineffective as well. The usual dose is 60 mg per day divided into two to three doses. Its side effects are very similar to those of verapamil.

- **BETA-BLOCKERS** are, at times, mildly effective for cluster patients, but much less effective generally than the usual cluster therapies. Propranolol (Inderal) or nadolol (Corgard) are discussed in Chapter 6.

- **MISCELLANEOUS ANTIDEPRESSANTS** (amitriptyline, Prozac, Zoloft, Paxil) are occasionally helpful, but usually not adequate by themselves. (See Chapter 6.)

- **LONG-ACTING DAILY OPIOIDS** (see Chapter 6) are more useful for severe chronic daily headache and migraines. If all else fails, though, they may be worthwhile for cluster headaches.

- **METHYLPHENIDATE (RITALIN)** may occasionally be effective in stopping a cluster in progress. Low doses (10 mg) are typical; 30 mg per day should be the limit. Side effects include anxiety, insomnia, fatigue, and addiction, among others.

ADDITIONAL TREATMENTS FOR PREVENTING CHRONIC CLUSTER HEADACHES

To prevent chronic cluster headaches, a doctor will probably use the same treatments as for episodic clusters. When nothing else seems effective and the pain is consistently on the same side, then the doctor may suggest a surgical technique conducted at only a few medical centers.

Radiofrequency trigeminal rhizotomy kills trigeminal nerve fibers involved in pain conduction, but sometimes the procedure must be repeated to be effective. A specialized technique, the surgery is conducted primarily at neurosurgery centers that specialize in pain treatment. A newer technique using "gamma knife radiation" is promising, and relatively noninvasive. These techniques are similar to those used for trigeminal neuralgia. Injections of botulinum toxin (Botox, et cetera) are promising for migraine and may help some cluster patients as well.

CASE STUDIES

As we have discussed, medication for clusters is used only during the cluster cycle and not in between. Abortive medication offers some relief once the clusters begin, and preventive medication helps avoid potentially disabling and excruciating pain. Here are several typical cluster headache cases.

RICHARD

INITIAL VISIT: Richard, a forty-year-old lawyer, has a five-year history of suffering from five weeks of cluster headaches each fall. The cluster period begins slowly, increasing over one week and reaching a peak in which Richard has two or three severe cluster attacks each day. They occur between ten P.M. and three A.M. and last forty to ninety minutes. The pain is always on the right side, with the eye tearing and right nostril congested.

He is now one week into his fall cluster series. The headaches are increasing in intensity, and he is miserable with the pain. Richard's doctor prescribes abortive medication to ease an attack in progress as well as a preventive regimen.

Richard and his doctor discuss using oxygen as an abortive, but Richard prefers to try Cafergot tablets first. He has no risk factors for ergotamines and is reluctant to self-inject DHE or sumatriptan. He will take one Cafergot at the beginning of the cluster and apply ice to the painful area.

For preventive therapy, the doctor prescribes 20 mg of prednisone (cortisone or corticosteroid) in the morning and 20 mg with dinner, or 40 mg per day for four days, to be reduced gradually over the next two weeks. By tapering this medication quickly, Richard avoids the risk of serious side effects and he can reserve the medication for use later in the cluster period, if necessary. If Richard were taking medium to high cortisone doses for three weeks, it would not be safe to use even more cortisone, so he keeps his use to a minimum.

Along with the cortisone, the doctor prescribes 240 mg of the calcium blocker verapamil, hoping that by the time the prednisone is tapered and discontinued, the verapamil will have become effective.

DAY 6: Richard reports that he had five very good days, but as the prednisone is decreased, the headaches become more severe. Cafergot does not help; last night he had ninety minutes of extreme pain. Richard now agrees to give oxygen a try and rents a tank. The doctor gives him a plastic spray bottle of topical lidocaine, 4 percent, to use as needed on the side of the pain. He is to lie supine, turn his head toward the side of the pain, extend it back, and spray two or three times into the nostril as needed. While lidocaine is only somewhat effective for cluster headaches, side effects are minimal. Even just 25 percent relief makes the lidocaine worthwhile. In addition, Richard is given Imitrex Nasal Spray to use as needed (applied on the opposite side of the pain).

Richard is to continue decreasing the prednisone, with a now doubled dose of verapamil (480 mg per day) to maintain the preventive therapy.

DAY 10: Now in the third week of what is expected to be a five-week cycle, Richard reports that the oxygen helps, but lidocaine does not. The clusters are less severe but continue to occur twice a night. The Imitrex Nasal Spray is only mildly effective. The verapamil may be having some effect. He is down to 20 mg per day of prednisone, and he and his doctor decide to taper off the prednisone over the next six days. If the headaches get dramatically worse, he can increase it again. Richard agrees to use Imitrex injections as needed.

DAY 14: Richard had complete relief for four days, and then the headaches returned but were not nearly as severe.

DAY 20: The headaches are gone, and after one week Richard tapers off the verapamil over six days. If the headaches return during those six days, he will increase the verapamil again, to 480 mg per day, and may reinstitute the prednisone.

THE FUTURE: The next time Richard's cluster period begins, he will use oxygen and Imitrex injections as abortives. He will begin taking verapamil and about two weeks' worth of prednisone. Lithium and Depakote are other possible preventives.

SHELDON

INITIAL VISIT: Sheldon is a fifty-five-year-old insurance salesman who has been getting episodic cluster headaches once or twice a year ever since he was twenty-six. They usually occur for six or eight weeks, in the spring and fall, with two to four headaches per twenty-four hours. The headaches are always around Sheldon's left eye, with tearing, running of the left nostril, and tenderness in the back of his head. The pain typically begins at ten or eleven P.M. and often awakens him from sleep. The headache lasts two hours and is sharp and extremely debilitating. Sheldon feels completely incapacitated during the headache cycle. His dad had migraines. Sheldon smokes cigarettes. Alcohol and MSG trigger increased headaches during the cluster cycle, but outside of the cycle, Sheldon never experiences a cluster headache.

Cortisone medication (Decadron, Medrol, prednisone) was effective for a number of years as a preventive used during the cluster period, but it no longer helps. Methysergide (Sansert) did not help, and verapamil (Isoptin, Calan) helped until last year, but is no longer effective. Other than smoking, Sheldon has no cardiac (heart) risk factors.

One week into the cluster series, Sheldon is placed on lithium, 600 mg (two pills), as a preventive medication to be taken at dinnertime because his headaches occur primarily at night. His doctor teaches him how to self-inject sumatriptan (Imitrex), which helps the vast majority of cluster sufferers. Imitrex is expensive, but it often stops the cluster pain within minutes. Sheldon also receives a small tank of oxygen, to breathe eight liters per minute, as needed, by mask. Sheldon is instructed to quit smoking gradually, as this often will cut down on the clusters.

WEEK 3: Sheldon reports that the clusters have decreased with the lithium, down to one every other night. The Imitrex does stop the clusters within ten minutes, but the oxygen helps only a little. Sheldon does not want to use Imitrex for every headache, so the doctor prescribes the butalbital compound Fiorinal as a pain reliever. While the analgesics, such as Fiorinal, are not ideal for treating clusters, they are useful at times. The pain pills do take at least twenty to thirty minutes to become effective.

WEEK 8: Sheldon reports that the lithium was helpful for four weeks but then ceased being effective. The dose is increased to three pills per day.

WEEK 9: The increased dose of lithium still does not help. The doctor prescribes Depakote, which is occasionally useful for clusters. Because Sheldon is fifty-five, Depakote is safer for him than daily ergotamines. If the Depakote is not effective, however, Sheldon's doctor might consider trying indomethacin (Indocin).

WEEK 10: The Depakote is not effective. Sheldon decides that because the headache cycle is due to end soon, he will simply use abortive medications — Imitrex injections, oxygen, and Fiorinal — and not pursue preventive measures.

THE FUTURE: When the next cycle begins, Indocin will be a very reasonable preventive alternative for Sheldon. The other medications have either stopped working or never worked for him. He will continue to take Fiorinal and Imitrex as abortives.

Imitrex Nasal Spray is a reasonable (but less effective) alternative to the injection. A steroid blockade of the occipital nerve (see the section earlier in this chapter) would also be a reasonable therapy.

11

· · · · · · · · ·

HEADACHES IN CHILDREN
AND ADOLESCENTS

WITNESSING your child endure the pain of headaches can be particularly difficult. For one thing, it is always hard to see your children in pain. In the case of headaches, you may feel guilty that something you did, such as arguing with them or with a spouse, may have contributed to their distress. Or you may get headaches yourself and worry that your child may develop a similar pattern. You may also feel helpless, not quite sure how you can aid your child in pain.

When your child has frequent headaches, it can be hard on the entire family. He or she may miss a lot of school, siblings may complain over the attention paid to the sick child, or the child may relish all the extra attention and then exaggerate the head pain to keep getting more. Adolescents who get severe, frequent headaches often become depressed, and that can affect the whole family, too.

Although headaches are difficult illnesses, especially in children, you can rest assured: many nondrug strategies can help prevent headaches in children, and when medication is needed to relieve pain and restore the quality of life, there is a safe and effective arsenal from which to draw.

WHO GETS HEADACHES?

Unfortunately, many children get headaches. Head pain accounts for more than a million lost days of school every year. Even

two-year-olds can get migraines, although they often are misdiagnosed as flu symptoms. Age six is a more typical time for migraines
to start, especially among boys. By age seven, some 40 percent of
children will have had a headache; most are minor tension (muscle
contraction) headaches. By age ten, 4 percent have had a migraine.
After age twelve, many boys outgrow childhood migraines, while
girls start getting more of them as their hormones change. All
told, about one in ten children and adolescents may suffer from
migraines.

SYMPTOMS IN CHILDREN

If your family has a history of migraines and your child gets severe
headaches, there is a good chance that they are inherited and that
they're migraines. Other clues leading to migraines are headaches
associated with nausea, visual auras, or typical migraine triggers,
such as particular foods or stress. The stress that triggers migraines may not always be "bad stress" but may be "good stress,"
such as the excitement of a birthday party or a special trip. Under-
sleeping also results in a headache.

Migraines in children may follow a different pattern from the
one they do in adults. For one, they tend to be shorter and often
begin with no warning, such as flashing lights or an aura. Also,
children often suffer from abdominal pain and diarrhea as well as
the typical adult symptoms, such as nausea and sensitivity to light.
The nausea often is severe in children and comes on early in the
migraine. And although adult migraines are usually concentrated
on one side of the head, children often experience pain on both
sides.

Tension headaches in children, on the other hand, tend to resemble tension headaches in adults. If the headaches are severe
and recurring, they are likely to be migraines and are treated as
such because distinguishing between a severe tension headache
and a mild migraine is very difficult, if not impossible.

If your child is getting severe or regular headaches, it is important to consult a doctor to rule out any physiological problems.

About one in twenty children with headache is not suffering from a tension or migraine headache, but from a neurological illness, hormonal dysfunctions, eye problems, meningitis, infection, or other potentially serious medical condition, even a viral infection from a bite from a pet mouse. Assuming that's not the case, the next step is to try to relieve the pain with nondrug strategies and over-the-counter medications, and, if possible, to identify and avoid headache triggers.

NONDRUG STRATEGIES TO PREVENT HEADACHES IN CHILDREN

Before we discuss how to avoid tension headaches and migraines — the two most common types of headaches in children — consider that some headaches in children are caused by eyestrain (too much TV or time before a computer monitor, a need for prescriptive eyeglasses) or an injury to the head. These factors may be involved when your child complains of headaches.

HEADACHE HELP TIP

If your child is getting frequent headaches, the first thing to do is to make sure that he or she doesn't need glasses or a stronger prescription. Also, consider too much TV or too much time in front of the computer screen as a possible cause.

IDENTIFYING AND AVOIDING TRIGGERS can be very effective in warding off migraines in children. These factors include certain foods, too little sleep, smoke and other fumes, weather changes, fatigue, stress, bright lights, hunger, heavy exercise, travel, and so on. We explore these triggers in detail in Chapter 6. In addition to the foods listed there, high-sugar and high-salt foods are also potential triggers in children. Restricting what your child eats can be difficult, especially if you need to eliminate favorite foods. Try to enlist your child's cooperation and experiment. He or she can either stop eating all the possible trigger foods at once, or a few at a time (the most common or likely suspects), adding them back one by one. Put together a chart and a calendar with your child; the more active your child is in maintaining these tools, the more cooperation will result.

RELAXATION AND BIOFEEDBACK techniques can be very effective with children as young as seven or eight who can learn the simple breathing and imaging techniques to deal with stress that could be triggering headaches. Children nine and older can learn the more complex adult techniques described in Chapter 2. Because children are sensitive to stress, consider whether your child's routine is too hectic. Medication in children should be minimal, so it is extremely important to explore these techniques fully. They can be very effective yet are tragically underused.

PEER GROUPS OR INDIVIDUAL COUNSELING is especially useful for adolescents and their parents. Many children and adolescents who get severe headaches drive themselves hard, insist on perfection, participate in many activities, are completely stressed out and prone to depression, and need to explore and share these issues with peers in a similar situation or with a psychotherapist. Talk to your child's doctor or guidance counselor. If there is not an appropriate group already in your area, think about starting one.

As children move into adolescence, stress in their lives gets more intense, and anxiety and depression become more common. Getting frequent headaches itself is a stressor.

Often, children need individual counseling and/or family therapy to learn better coping skills and to express feelings and thoughts that are bottled up inside. Although biofeedback and relaxation therapies can be useful to children, psychotherapy and family therapy can have even more dramatic positive results.

Some children have so many headaches that they miss weeks, months, or even years of school. Many miss fifty, even sixty days a year. Therapy in almost all these cases is appropriate and necessary if the headaches are to be treated effectively.

RELIEVING HEADACHES IN CHILDREN
UNDER AGE ELEVEN

Once headaches start, the fairly simple methods that follow can relieve the vast majority. If the child is older than eleven, the strategies shift toward the management techniques for adults. We'll address specific adolescent concerns later in this chapter.

At the first sign of a headache, either migraine or tension, get your child comfortable in a dark, quiet room and apply ice to his head. Consult with the doctor about experimenting with limited amounts of acetaminophen or ibuprofen and perhaps some caffeine.

QUICK REFERENCE GUIDE

FIRST-LINE MEDICATIONS

FOR CHILDREN'S HEADACHES

OVER-THE-COUNTER

1. ACETAMINOPHEN (TYLENOL AND SIMILAR PRODUCTS)
   Mild and safe; add some caffeine with cola, for example.

2. IBUPROFEN (MOTRIN, ADVIL, NUPRIN)
   Stronger, but higher incidence of stomach problems.

3. CAFFEINE
   Good either by itself (cola, caffeine gum, pills) or with the above medications.

PRESCRIPTION

1. NAPROXEN (ALEVE, NAPROSYN, ANAPROX)
   Stronger than OTC medications but sometimes cause stomachaches. Add caffeine. Aleve is OTC.

2. MIDRIN
   Used when the above medications don't help; these are big capsules but can be emptied into food.

SECOND-LINE MEDICATIONS
FOR CHILDREN'S HEADACHES

1. BUTALBITAL COMPOUNDS
　　Very effective but a sedative.

2. ASPIRIN
　　Effective, but avoid if child has chicken pox or the flu with a fever. Adding caffeine helps.

THIRD-LINE MEDICATIONS
FOR CHILDREN'S HEADACHES

1. PREDNISONE
　　Strong medication that's used to break the cycle of many migraines.

2. MIGRANAL (DHE) NASAL SPRAY AND INJECTIONS
　　Sometimes the only thing that will work; IV most effective.

3. TRIPTANS (IMITREX, MAXALT, AMERGE, ZOMIG, RELPAX)
　　For children over nine, low doses can be helpful.

FIRST-LINE MEDICATIONS FOR
RELIEVING HEADACHES IN CHILDREN

1. ACETAMINOPHEN

Acetaminophen, the medication used in Tylenol, is well tolerated, safe, and has few side effects, but it is not as effective as ibuprofen or aspirin. Because it is safe, however, acetaminophen is usually the first medication children should try. Giving the child some caffeine, such as cola, can enhance the drug's effectiveness. Chewable tablets, liquid, and suppository forms are available.

ASPIRIN-FREE EXCEDRIN combines acetaminophen with 65 mg of caffeine and is more useful for migraine than for daily headache. Children often need to be at least nine to tolerate this dose of caffeine.

TYPICAL DOSE: When calculated by weight, the dose is approximately 3 to 5 mg per pound (5 to 10 mg per kg) every two to four hours (maximum per day of 15 or 20 mg per pound or 30 or 40 mg per kg). Three doses in twenty-four hours at most.

By age, rather than weight, typical doses are 240 mg per dose for four- and five-year-olds, 320 mg per dose for six- to eight-year-olds, 400 mg for nine- and ten-year-olds, and 480 mg per dose for eleven-year-olds. Three doses per twenty-four hours should be the maximum. If your child needs more than one dose a day, *every day*, however, consider preventive medication.

Acetaminophen is available in many forms, including chewable tablets in 80, 120, and 160 mg; regular (nonchewable) tablets in 325, 500, and 650 mg; capsules in 325 or 500 mg; and syrup in concentrations of 80, 120, 160, and 325 mg per teaspoon. There is also a Tylenol Extra-Strength liquid with 500 mg per three teaspoons.

Suppositories are available in strengths of 120, 125, 325, 600, and 650 mg. Finally, there is a fizzy antacid with buffered acetaminophen that contains 325 mg per three-quarters of a cap, as well as sodium bicarbonate and citric acid.

SIDE EFFECTS: Rare. Occasional fatigue.

2. IBUPROFEN

Ibuprofen is the generic chemical used in Advil, Motrin, and Nuprin, among others. It is more effective for migraines and tension headaches than acetaminophen but poses a greater risk of causing gastrointestinal upset, nausea, fatigue, and dizziness. Nevertheless, it is generally well tolerated. Again, giving your child caffeine in some form can enhance the drug's effectiveness. Liquid Advil is useful for younger children.

TYPICAL DOSE: Ages four to five, 100 mg (one teaspoon of the Children's Advil liquid) every three to four hours, as needed; ages six to eight, 100 to 150 mg (one to one and a half teaspoons) every three to four hours, as needed; ages nine to ten, 150 to

200 mg per dose; ages eleven to twelve, 200 to 400 mg per dose. Three doses per day at most. Maximum daily dose is 15 mg per pound (30 mg per kg) per day.

3. CAFFEINE

Caffeine can be used by itself (in a cola drink or in pill form) or with acetaminophen or ibuprofen. It can help either a tension or a migraine headache. When used in limited amounts, its side effects are minimal.

FIRST-LINE PRESCRIPTION MEDICATIONS FOR TREATING HEADACHES IN CHILDREN

When the simpler combinations of acetaminophen, ibuprofen, and caffeine aren't powerful enough to help your child, you'll probably need to identify with your child's doctor a stronger abortive medication to relieve a headache in progress. In the vast majority of cases with children, a good abortive is all that you'll need. However, if the abortive needs to be used more than three times a week or the headaches are sporadic but severe (and therefore usually considered migraines), the doctor may recommend a preventive medication.

As we discuss in other chapters, many medications helpful for headache have not received specific approval from the FDA for headache or for children. You should fully understand the risks, side effects, and problems associated with any medication before you give it to your child. Check a medication reference book or the package insert. Any discussion of medications here is for information, not a suggestion for use. Only a physician who knows your child's individual situation can make an informed recommendation.

If you know from experience that you will want to give the child an abortive medication if a headache starts, do so as early as possible to make it most effective. If the child is nauseated, either wait for the nausea to subside or for the child to vomit, and then use the abortive medication, or consider an antinausea medication. Rectal suppositories for combating nausea are more effective than oral medication and more useful when oral medications are not well tolerated; many children, however, feel too embarrassed to use them. Remember also that almost all of the medications listed in this chapter may be formulated by pharmacists into flavored lozenges for children who cannot swallow pills or are too nauseated to swallow medication.

If your child is ten or younger and a combination of caffeine, acetaminophen, and ibuprofen doesn't work, your doctor will probably recommend one of these medications.

1. NAPROXEN (ALEVE, NAPROSYN, ANAPROX)

More effective than acetaminophen or ibuprofen, naproxen does often cause temporary gastrointestinal distress. Sedation also occasionally occurs. Its liquid form can be particularly useful for children. Having a small amount of caffeine with naproxen can usually enhance its effectiveness. A lower-dose naproxen tablet (Aleve, 220 mg) is available over the counter but should be used only under a doctor's supervision, as is true for all prescription medications.

If used daily, kidney and liver functions need be monitored.

TYPICAL DOSE: For a fifty-pound child, one teaspoon, or 125 mg, to start; may be repeated once per day. For an eighty-five-pound child, one to one and a half teaspoons, or 125 to about 185 mg per dose; may be repeated once only. For a child one hundred pounds or more, 275 mg of Anaprox or 250 mg of naproxen or 220 mg of Aleve.

2. MIDRIN

Usually Midrin is recommended when neither the over-the-counter medications nor naproxen works well. This medication, available in capsule form, consists of acetaminophen, a mild vasoconstrictor (isometheptene mucate), and a nonaddicting sedative (dichloralphenazone). The large capsules may be taken apart and emptied into applesauce or juice (the capsule shell itself does not need to be swallowed). Midrin tends to be reasonably effective and may be used in children as young as age seven. (See Chapter 5 for more details.)

TYPICAL DOSE: For ages seven and eight, a quarter or half capsule, repeated every two hours if necessary but limited to two full capsules in one day. For ages nine and ten, a half or whole capsule, repeated if necessary at two-hour intervals, three in one day at the most.

SIDE EFFECTS: Sedation and lightheadedness, occasional stomach upset.

If these first-line medications are ineffective or inappropriate for your child, the doctor may then recommend:

SECOND-LINE MEDICATIONS FOR TREATING HEADACHES IN CHILDREN

1. BUTALBITAL COMPOUNDS

These medications are generally well tolerated and extremely effective. The butalbital is a sedative, which in most cases is useful to help the child sleep away the headache.

Fiorinal (which contains aspirin) is more effective than Esgic or Fioricet (which contains acetaminophen and caffeine), which, in turn, is more effective than Phrenilin (acetaminophen but no caffeine). See Chapter 5 for more information.

• FIORINAL

Fiorinal contains 50 mg of the short-acting sedative butalbital, 325 mg of aspirin, and 40 mg of caffeine, which helps offset the sedative. The tablets may be cut in half for children. Because of the aspirin component, this medication must be used with caution to avoid the risk of Reye's syndrome, a disease of the brain, marked by fever, vomiting, and swelling of the kidneys and brain.

TYPICAL DOSE: For ages seven and eight, half a tablet, which may be repeated within an hour or two, but daily maximum should be no more than one tablet per day. For ages nine and ten, a half or whole tablet, which may be repeated in three hours, with a maximum of two tablets in one day.

SIDE EFFECTS: Fatigue and sometimes nervousness; nausea or gastrointestinal pain from the aspirin; lightheadedness, dizziness, or euphoria from the butalbital.

- **ESGIC, FIORICET**

These medications, which are identical except that Esgic is available in capsule or pill form and Fioricet only in pill form, are less effective than Fiorinal but better tolerated because they contain acetaminophen rather than aspirin. They consist of 50 mg of butalbital, 325 mg of acetaminophen, and 40 mg of caffeine. Since the brand name medications are usually more effective the generic is best avoided.

TYPICAL DOSE: Same as for Fiorinal.

SIDE EFFECTS: Fatigue, occasional nervousness; nausea but less so than with Fiorinal. Lightheadedness, dizziness, and euphoria may occur.

- **PHRENILIN**

Phrenilin (50 mg of butalbital and 325 mg of acetaminophen) is the same as Esgic but has no caffeine. It is particularly helpful for children who cannot take caffeine or aspirin.

TYPICAL DOSE: Same as for Fiorinal.

SIDE EFFECTS: Usually mild, though sedation is very common. Lightheadedness, dizziness, and euphoria may occur.

2. ASPIRIN

Although aspirin is quite effective and well tolerated, it is not a first choice because of the fear, founded or unfounded, of Reye's syndrome. However, unless a child has chicken pox or the flu with fever, aspirin is a safe bet. Nevertheless, many parents are reluctant to use aspirin in any situation.

Taking aspirin with caffeinated soda can relieve pain even more.

TYPICAL DOSE: For ages six to eight, 325 mg three times a day. For ages nine to ten, 400 mg three times a day, at most. Children's aspirin is available in 65, 75, and 81 mg tablets, and in 81 mg chewable tablets. Aspergum (chewing gum) has 227.5 mg each. Standard aspirin is 325 mg per tablet.

SIDE EFFECTS: Gastrointestinal upset.

When none of the first- or second-line medications is useful and your child continues to suffer from severe, prolonged headaches, which will probably be diagnosed as migraines, your doctor may recommend Prednisone or DHE. When prescribed for children, these drugs are used in very limited doses and for very short periods of time. Also remember that you can ask a pharmacist to formulate these medications into lozenges.

THIRD-LINE MEDICATIONS FOR TREATING HEADACHES IN CHILDREN

1. PREDNISONE

Prednisone becomes useful when your child is enduring a prolonged pattern of migraines that have been resistant to other medications. It should be able to break the painful cycle. Occasionally, small doses of Decadron, a corticosteroid (see Chapter 5), may be used instead.

TYPICAL DOSE: Usually 10 mg by mouth twice a day, with food, as needed, for one or two days only; 40 mg total per migraine. If the headache is relieved with smaller doses, then medication should be stopped.

SIDE EFFECTS: In these small doses, side effects are minimal. Anxiety or gastrointestinal upset are the most common. Fatigue, insomnia, and dizziness may also occur.

2. MIGRANAL (DHE) NASAL SPRAY AND INJECTIONS (FOR AGES NINE AND OLDER)

DHE is sometimes the only medication that effectively relieves a severe and prolonged migraine. Administering this medication intravenously is more effective, less painful, and better tolerated by children than intramuscular injections. The Migranal Nasal Spray is well tolerated.

NASAL SPRAY TYPICAL DOSE: One spray in one nostril once every thirty minutes, two sprays total in one day at most.

INJECTION TYPICAL DOSE: One-time dose of 0.3 to 0.5 mg intravenously. When the migraine is severe and resistant to other therapies, a second dose may be given.

SIDE EFFECTS: Nausea, lightheadedness, a feeling of heat about the head, muscle contraction headaches, and leg cramps may occur. Migranal may cause stuffiness of the nose.

(See Chapter 5 for a detailed discussion of this medication.)

3. Triptans (Imitrex, Maxalt, Amerge, Zomig, Relpax)

Although not officially approved by the FDA for children, the triptans are occasionally used for children nine or older. Very low doses are used — half a tablet only, or the low-dose 5-mg Imitrex Nasal Spray.

ANTINAUSEA MEDICATIONS FOR CHILDREN

As we mentioned previously, many children get nauseated with a migraine, especially early in the headache. It is usually better to let children throw up and then give them an abortive medication to ease the pain. If they can't keep the medication down, then try an antinausea medication. Unfortunately, there sometimes is little choice but to use a suppository (although a pharmacist may be able to formulate a flavored lozenge for you). These medications not only ease nausea, but in some cases, such as with promethazine, they will sedate the child, thereby helping to relieve the migraine.

Trimethobenzamide (Tigan) or promethazine (Phenergan) are the most commonly prescribed antinausea medications for children. They are detailed in Chapter 5. Other, more effective medications, such as prochlorperazine (Compazine), cause more disturbing side effects, such as anxiety, in children.

1. Trimethobenzamide (Tigan)

Tigan is extremely well tolerated, which is why it is so commonly used in children.

TYPICAL DOSE: 100 to 200 mg every four hours as needed to relieve nausea. Available in capsules, suppositories, syrups, and injections, or may be formulated as a flavored lozenge by a compounding pharmacist.

SIDE EFFECTS: Fatigue. Low blood pressure (hypotension), confusion, blurred vision, disorientation, muscle cramps, and dizziness occasionally occur.

2. Promethazine (Phenergan)

Phenergan is also well tolerated and often causes sedation, which may be desired.

TYPICAL DOSE: 12.5 to 25 mg per dose, or 0.15 to 0.25 per pound (0.25 to 0.5 mg per kg per dose), which may be repeated if necessary; three doses per day is the usual maximum. Available in tablets, syrup, suppositories, or injection. Flavored oral lozenges may be formulated by a compounding pharmacist.

SIDE EFFECTS: Sedation, which is helpful for relieving pain by inducing sleep. Low blood pressure (hypotension), blurred vision, disorientation, and dizziness may occur but are not common.

PREVENTING HEADACHES IN CHILDREN UNDER AGE ELEVEN

If biofeedback and nonmedication therapies have been earnestly tried to no avail and your child is taking an abortive medication frequently and still getting more than three or four moderate to severe migraines in a typical month, your doctor may recommend preventive medication.

When considering a preventive, be prepared to use it daily and expect the possibility of some side effects as well as the potential need to change medications if one doesn't prove effective or causes severe side effects. Preventive medication in children and adolescents should be kept to a minimum and stopped periodically. As with adults, the goal is to return to abortive medications exclusively if possible.

For children younger than age eleven, the medications used to prevent migraines tend to be the same as for chronic (tension) daily headache, so they are not separated out here unless indicated.

QUICK REFERENCE GUIDE:
PREVENTING HEADACHES IN CHILDREN

1. CYPROHEPTADINE (PERIACTIN)
An antihistamine that's inexpensive, safe, and sometimes useful.

2. NSAIDs (IBUPROFEN, NAPROXEN)
Can be very effective and don't cause sedation, cognitive changes, or decreased energy level.

3. PROPRANOLOL (INDERAL)
A beta-blocker that's often useful for migraines but not daily headaches. Fatigue and stomach problems are fairly common.

4. ANTIDEPRESSANTS
Good for daily headaches because they affect serotonin levels; can have numerous side effects, from fatigue and sedation to a dry mouth, weight gain, and insomnia.

PRESCRIPTION MEDICATIONS FOR PREVENTING HEADACHES IN CHILDREN

1. CYPROHEPTADINE (PERIACTIN)

This medication, an antihistamine often prescribed for allergies, also influences serotonin. It is inexpensive and safe, though it is not always the most effective choice. It tends to be most useful for children ten years old and younger. Because it may be taken just once a day and in liquid form, it can be quite convenient.

TYPICAL DOSE: 4 mg per day, tablet or liquid, taken at night; doses may be gradually increased to as high as 12 mg, as needed. Larger doses are split for twice-a-day dosing.

SIDE EFFECTS: Fatigue and weight gain due to increased appetite.

2. NSAIDs (Ibuprofen, Naproxen)

A daily anti-inflammatory can be very effective in preventing headaches and may be preferred to the other preventives because it has no effect on energy level, sedation, or cognitive functions (memory or concentration problems). Its doses should be kept to a minimum and, with blood tests performed periodically, long-term use can be quite safe. NSAIDs have been used safely for years, for example, for juvenile rheumatoid arthritis in doses much higher than used for headaches.

TYPICAL DOSE: For ibuprofen, at age five, half a teaspoon of the 100 mg syrup, or 50 mg per day. At ages six to eight, the dose is half to one teaspoon, or 50 to 100 mg per day. At ages nine to ten, the dose increases to one or two teaspoons, or 100 to 200 mg per day. The regular tablets are 200 mg.

Naproxen doses are calculated by weight, half to one teaspoon daily. One teaspoon is equal to half of the 250 mg pill. (See "First-Line Prescription Medications for Treating Headaches in Children" for more details.) Over-the-counter Aleve dose is 220 mg.

3. Propranolol (Inderal)

This beta-blocker that prevents blood vessel dilation is quite effective for migraines but only occasionally effective for daily headaches. It is very well tolerated but should not be taken by asthmatic children.

TYPICAL DOSE: 0.5 to 1.0 mg per pound per day (or 1 to 2 mg per kg per day), starting with a low dose and increasing it if necessary. The long-acting capsule cannot be divided.

SIDE EFFECTS: Fatigue and lower abdominal upset are fairly common. Less common is a decrease in heart rate and blood pressure, with a corresponding decrease in stamina. Memory or concentration difficulties, dizziness, and lightheadedness may occur.

4. Antidepressants

Because of their effects on serotonin, antidepressants, such as amitriptyline (Elavil), nortriptyline (Pamelor, Aventyl), or SSRIs (Prozac, Zoloft, Paxil), are a first-choice medication for moderate to severe chronic daily headaches. They are usually not prescribed for migraines, however, until cyproheptadine and the NSAIDs have been tried.

Amitriptyline and nortriptyline are similar medications, except that amitriptyline is less expensive and tends to be somewhat more effective. Nortriptyline, however, tends to have fewer side effects. (For a fuller discussion of amitriptyline and nortriptyline, see Chapters 6 and 9 on preventive medications for migraines and tension headaches in adults.)

TYPICAL DOSE: The SSRIs (selective serotonin reuptake inhibitors, such as Prozac, Zoloft, Paxil) have been proven safe for children and adolescents. They may be safer, in fact, than the older (tricyclic) antidepressants. Low doses are used for headaches, 10 mg to start, usually at night, increased if necessary to 25 or 50 mg (occasionally up to 75 or 100 mg). The average dose in this age range is 25 mg. For the SSRIs, starting doses are low, such as 5 mg of Prozac, 25 mg of Zoloft, or 5 mg of Paxil.

SIDE EFFECTS: Fatigue, sedation, anxiety, weight gain, a dry mouth, and dizziness; insomnia and memory or concentration difficulties may follow; occasional rapid heartbeat and blurred vision. These side effects are much more common with amitriptylene or nortriptyline than with the SSRIs (Prozac, Zoloft, Paxil).

RELIEVING HEADACHES IN ADOLESCENTS OVER AGE ELEVEN

After age ten, many boys "outgrow" bad headache spells, and girls end up having headache woes about three times more often than boys do. Both tension and migraine are problems among adolescents.

As children plow their way through the stormy and highly stressful teen years, anxiety and depression become increasingly common. Teenagers feel a lot of stress and pressure, including pressure from and conflicts with parents, peer pressure, anxiety from coping with their new bodies, new kinds of relationships, and new kinds of responsibilities. All these factors can exacerbate headaches. To make matters worse, when headaches are not well controlled, just having the headaches intensifies feelings of stress, anxiety, and depression. Some research suggests that adolescents who get frequent headaches are more likely to be "Type A" personalities — hard-driving perfectionists with quick tempers.

Individual counseling or family therapy can be crucial to improving how a teenager copes with stress and depression, which, in turn, can dramatically relieve the frequency and intensity of headaches. Although many teenagers are reluctant to discuss their problems with parents or physicians, many respond very well to a sympathetic therapist. Adolescents also should be encouraged to learn relaxation techniques, such as deep breathing and biofeedback. Stress is a major trigger in this age range, and looking at stressors is crucial. Many studies have indicated that in adolescence, particularly with daily or frequent tension headaches, there is a high chance of finding anxiety or hidden depression or both. A good psychotherapist can be crucial in helping to improve the situation both through counseling and teaching relaxation techniques.

Help your teen use other self-help techniques, such as avoiding trigger foods, not missing meals, and getting enough sleep (most adolescents need eight to ten hours; they rarely get enough and almost always go to bed too late).

A small group of kids miss weeks, months, or even years of school because of head pain. Typically, these adolescents and their families have complex issues to confront, and physicians have been remarkably unsuccessful in helping their headaches without counseling. In general, a "tough-love" approach, with virtually no excuse accepted for missing school, is usually best. Nevertheless, a few adolescents do fare better with home tutoring.

The goal with adolescents is to help the headaches, but minimize medications. Although most adolescents don't need preventive medication, many do need abortive medication to relieve a headache in progress. During periods of severe or frequent headaches, however, daily preventive medication may be necessary on a temporary basis. Preventive medication may also be called for if your teen chases after headaches all day with abortive medications, which can trigger rebound headaches. Occasionally, adolescents might also use a daily preventive medication if they are anxious or depressed, or if they have trouble sleeping.

Tension and migraine headaches are treated similarly in teens, except that migraine sufferers often need an antinausea medication as well. Teens take the same medications as children do, except that they may use aspirin more readily and may be able to tolerate some stronger medications. Because we have detailed all these medications elsewhere, we simply list them here to indicate the order in which they are usually prescribed for adolescents, as well as their most prominent features and the most typical doses for teenagers. These doses tend to be the same as the low-range doses for adults. As always, these medications should be taken with food.

In general, doctors use daily anti-inflammatories for this age range (the ibuprofen/Aleve type of medications) because they do not cause sedation or cognitive problems, such as "spaciness" or memory problems. Although the anti-inflammatories are associated with a high rate of stomach problems, this age group usually experiences fewer stomach problems with these medications than do other age groups. In general, the younger the person, the safer the anti-inflammatories; however, they can cause ulcers in any age.

MEDICATIONS FOR
TREATING HEADACHES IN ADOLESCENTS

Begin with these medications to try to relieve tension headaches in your adolescent. Note that they may also be effective for migraines, which we will discuss in the next section. The first four groups of medications are over-the-counter.

1. ACETAMINOPHEN
Best tolerated, least effective. Commonly known as Tylenol. Typical dose: 325 to 650 mg every four to six hours, as needed. Limit to 1,300 mg per day at most.

2. IBUPROFEN

More effective than acetaminophen but causes more side effects, especially stomach upset. Typical dose: 200 or 400 mg every four to six hours, as needed. Take with food. Taking with small amounts of caffeine may enhance effectiveness. Limit to 1200 mg in one day.

3. NAPROXEN (ALEVE, NAPROSYN, ANAPROX)

Widely used in adolescents, but stomach upset is common. Typical dose: For Aleve, 220-mg tablet every eight hours: for Naprosyn, 250-mg pill every eight hours. Taking with caffeine may help. Older adolescents may take two Aleve at a time.

4. ASPIRIN, ASPIRIN-FREE EXCEDRIN, ANACIN, EXCEDRIN EXTRA-STRENGTH, EXCEDRIN MIGRAINE

- **ASPIRIN**
  Typical dose: 325 mg every four to six hours, as needed.
- **ASPIRIN-FREE EXCEDRIN**
  Typical dose: one tablet every four to six hours, as needed.
- **ANACIN (ASPIRIN AND CAFFEINE)**
  Stomach upset is common and nervousness may occur. Typical dose: one Anacin tablet every four to six hours, as needed.
- **EXCEDRIN EXTRA-STRENGTH, EXCEDRIN MIGRAINE (ACETAMINOPHEN, ASPIRIN, AND CAFFEINE)**
  Most effective medication in this group but causes more side effects, such as rebound headaches, gastrointestinal upset, and nervousness. Typical dose: one tablet every four to six hours, as needed. For older adolescents, two tablets at the onset of a migraine may be effective.

5. NORGESIC FORTE (ASPIRIN, CAFFEINE, AND AN ANTIHISTAMINE, ORPHENADRINE CITRATE, WITH MUSCLE RELAXANT PROPERTIES)

Strong but nonaddicting. Typical dose: half to one pill every four hours, as needed, two in a day at most. Side effects include nervousness, drowsiness, a dry mouth, and stomach irritation because of the large amount of aspirin (770 mg aspirin per tablet).

6. KETOPROFEN (OrudisKT, GENERIC KETOPROFEN)

OrudisKT (or the generic) is a low-dose (12.5 mg) anti-inflammatory, useful for tension and migraine headaches. Typical dose: two tablets every three to four hours, with food. Stomach irritation may occur, as with the other anti-inflammatories. Taking with caffeine may help.

MEDICATIONS FOR TREATING MIGRAINE HEADACHES IN ADOLESCENTS

All these medications are discussed at length in Chapter 5.

1. TRIPTANS (IMITREX, ZOMIG, MAXALT, AMERGE, RELPAX)

While not officially indicated for use in adolescents, the triptans have been widely used in this age group. Low doses (half a tablet) are usually used first, but most adolescents require the usual adult dose. The side effects follow the same pattern as in adults.

2. MIDRIN

Especially good for migraines. Typical dose: One capsule (two may be needed at onset), repeated every two hours if needed; daily maximum dose is four or five capsules. Fatigue and dizziness are common.

3. BUTALBITAL COMPOUNDS (FIORINAL, FIORICET, ESGIC, PHRENILIN)

Habit-forming. Typical dose: Varies by medication but typically between the child and adult doses. Must be limited and not used more than one or two days per week.

4. OVER-THE-COUNTER ANTI-INFLAMMATORIES (IBUPROFEN, NAPROXEN, AND ASPIRIN [MOTRIN, ALEVE, AND BAYER, RESPECTIVELY], AS WELL AS EXCEDRIN EXTRA-STRENGTH AND EXCEDRIN MIGRAINE)

See Chapter 2 and Chapter 5 for detailed discussions.

5. Migranal (DHE) Nasal Spray

Well tolerated, Migranal is safe and effective. See the previous section in this chapter and also Chapter 5.

PREVENTING HEADACHES IN ADOLESCENTS OVER AGE ELEVEN

As with adults, psychotherapy or biofeedback can help some adolescents a great deal. But others who chase pain frequently with abortive medications, which can cause rebound headaches, will need a daily preventive for moderate or severe headaches.

When choosing preventives for this age range, the goal is to:

- minimize medications
- treat any concurrent conditions (such as depression or anxiety)
- get the adolescent off medications as quickly as possible — many do outgrow the headaches.

Since patterns of tension and migraine headaches are more prominent in teenagers than in younger children, the treatments do differ somewhat, as they do in adults. One major difference, however, is that as children become adolescents, the anti-inflammatories become a first-choice preventive for chronic daily headaches because they are so well tolerated by this age group. Again, these medications are detailed elsewhere, and we list them here in order of preference. The doses fall between those recommended for children and adults and will vary depending upon your teen's age and weight.

MEDICATIONS FOR PREVENTING TENSION HEADACHES IN ADOLESCENTS

(See Chapter 6 and Chapter 9 for detailed discussions.)

1. ANTI-INFLAMMATORIES: (IBUPROFEN, NAPROXEN, AND KETOPROFEN)

Very well tolerated and often effective, though they may cause stomach upset. Ibuprofen is relatively short acting and so is not ideal as a preventive medication. Ketoprofen is available over the counter as OrudisKT or as a once-daily prescription capsule (Oruvail).

2. ANTIDEPRESSANTS: SSRIs (PROZAC, PAXIL, ZOLOFT), NORTRIPTYLINE (PAMELOR, AVENTYL), PROTRIPTYLINE (VIVACTIL), AMITRIPTYLINE (ELAVIL)

These are the most effective preventives for migraines and daily headaches, but they cause more side effects (memory and concentration problems, a dry mouth, and dizziness are common) than the anti-inflammatories. Usually well tolerated in low doses and safe for long-term use. The SSRIs are generally much better tolerated than the older antidepressants. (See Chapters 6 and 9.)

3. VALPROATE (DEPAKOTE)

Extensively used for both migraine and tension headaches, Depakote has become a first-line medication for adolescents and adults. Low doses are used for adolescents. Side effects include weight gain, nausea, or fatigue.

MEDICATIONS FOR PREVENTING MIGRAINES IN ADOLESCENTS

If your adolescent is getting more than four migraines a month or if the migraines are very severe and fairly regular, the doctor will probably recommend preventive therapy. Sometimes preventive medication is even recommended for as little as one or two migraines per month if they are very severe and disruptive. The goal, as always, is to decrease frequency or severity by at least 70 percent, with as little medication as possible.

The first choices for preventing migraines in adolescents, in order of preference, are as follows:

1. ANTI-INFLAMMATORIES
The first choices, as they are for tension headaches.

2. VERAPAMIL (ISOPTIN, CALAN, VERELAN)
Often a good choice. Generally well tolerated, but constipation is common.

3. ANTIDEPRESSANTS
Highly effective. Tricyclics are the older antidepressants, such as amitriptyline, as opposed to the newer ones, like Prozac, Zoloft, and Paxil.

4. BETA-BLOCKERS

5. VALPROATE (DEPAKOTE)
Very effective for migraine and tension headaches.

If these first-line drugs prove ineffective or inappropriate, your doctor may suggest one of the following second-line choices:

1. COMBINING TWO OF THE FIRST- OR SECOND-LINE MEDICATIONS

2. FEVERFEW
This herb is relatively safe and has been proven to help prevent migraine headaches. It is usually well tolerated. (See Chapter 14.)

3. GABAPENTIN (NEURONTIN)
Related to Depakote, well tolerated, and generally safe. Tiredness is relatively common.

The third-line choices for preventing migraines in teens are:

1. PHENELZINE (NARDIL)

An MAO inhibitor.

2. INTRAVENOUS DHE

Please refer to previous chapters for details on all these medications.

CASE STUDIES

Here are some fairly typical cases among children and adolescents with migraines or tension headaches.

MEREDITH

INITIAL VISIT: Meredith is a nine-year-old with a history of migraines, twice a month, ever since she was six. The migraines last five hours, with a severe but short bout of nausea. Under-sleeping and chocolate are the only consistent triggers for Meredith's migraines. She also gets tension headaches, which occur three or four times a week and tend to worsen with stress. They usually occur toward the end of the school day and decrease in the summer.

Meredith's doctor teaches her basic deep-breathing–relaxation techniques, as age nine is a good time to try these methods. Meredith learns how to apply reusable ice packs to her head. Tylenol has been effective for her tension headaches, and she takes three or four chewable Tylenol tablets a week. Caffeine, in Coke or Pepsi, also helps. Meredith learns all of the usual migraine avoidance techniques, such as eating a diet that avoids trigger foods and wearing dark sunglasses on bright days.

WEEK 2: Meredith's mother reports that the deep-breathing–relaxation techniques are helping to relieve the tension headaches, but Meredith is still getting migraines. The doctor writes a prescription for liquid ibuprofen (Children's Advil), as Meredith has a difficult time swallowing tablets.

WEEK 4:   The ibuprofen helps relieve the migraine pain somewhat but increases her nausea. Meredith receives a prescription for liquid promethazine (Phenergan) for the nausea.

WEEK 16:   The ibuprofen is no longer effective, but the liquid Phenergan helps relieve the nausea. Meredith's doctor prescribes Midrin for the migraine pain and shows Meredith and her mother how to pull apart the capsule and put the powder in juice or applesauce.

WEEK 19:   The Phenergan and Midrin are sedating Meredith but are helping to reduce the pain by about 80 percent. Meredith wishes to try a medication that won't make her so sleepy. The Midrin is discontinued, and Meredith tries liquid Naprosyn, an anti-inflammatory similar to ibuprofen, instead.

WEEK 22:   The Naprosyn helps the pain about 60 percent and does not sedate Meredith. Although it increases her nausea, the Phenergan is controlling it. The plan is now for Meredith to use the Phenergan-Naprosyn combination if she's in school with pain, but if she's at home with a migraine, she'll use Phenergan with Midrin, which is more effective but puts her to sleep. Such a choice is not unusual for headache patients. They learn to use different medications in different situations.

THE FUTURE: If Meredith needs a change of medication, her doctor may prescribe a pure migraine medication, such as Migranal Nasal Spray. Butalbital medications, such as Fiorinal, Fioricet, Esgic, or Phrenilin, may also be helpful for Meredith at some point. Sedatives, such as diazepam (Valium), or narcotics, such as codeine, occasionally are useful in children of Meredith's age but are not generally used until other alternatives have been exhausted. Triptans, such as Imitrex, have occasionally been used for children at ages nine and ten.

MICHAEL

INITIAL VISIT: Michael, an eleven-year-old boy, has had monthly migraines since he was eight. Six months ago, he started to get moderately severe daily headaches. The migraines are also moderate to severe, last eight hours, and usually stop when he falls asleep. Michael vomits early in the migraine and then feels better. He becomes carsick easily, which is common among children with migraines. There is a strong family history of migraines, as both his mother and father have had migraines in the past. Michael does well in school and is a hard-driving perfectionist.

Acetaminophen or ibuprofen is only slightly effective for Michael's migraines. Caffeinated soft drinks do help to some degree. For the monthly migraine, Michael's doctor prescribes Midrin. Michael empties the contents of the large capsule into applesauce. He puts ice packs on his head as well.

The chronic daily headaches are more of a burden to Michael than the migraines. They last most of the day, every day. Occasionally, we find that children with headaches are "over-programmed" and under too much stress. While the headaches are worse with stress, they are also present when Michael is relaxed and on vacation. He and the doctor practice deep-breathing and relaxation techniques. After some discussion with Michael's parents, they decide to decrease his activities so that he does not have a planned activity day after day.

WEEK 2: The Midrin helps Michael's migraine, as do the ice packs, but makes him sedated and lightheaded. His doctor prescribes Migranal Nasal Spray instead of Midrin to help relieve any migraine. His daily headaches remain as bad as ever, and the doctor prescribes naproxen as a preventive medication, 220 mg per day.

WEEK 4: Michael's mother calls to say that the naproxen is working well to prevent the daily headaches, but that Michael had a migraine yesterday and the Migranal made him very sick. The doctor calls in a prescription to the pharmacy for Fioricet (acetaminophen, caffeine, and the mild sedative butalbital) to replace the Migranal.

WEEK 20: Michael comes in to the doctor's office and reports that he has felt better for several months, but his daily headaches are back. Evidently, the naproxen has lost its effectiveness. The doctor prescribes a low dose of amitriptyline (Elavil), 10 mg, to be taken at night.

WEEK 21: Michael's mother calls to say the medication seems to have no effect. The dose is raised to 25 mg.

WEEK 22: Michael's mother calls to say that the daily headaches have eased somewhat, but she would like to try a higher dose. The amitriptyline dose is raised to 50 mg.

WEEK 24: Michael's daily headaches have vastly improved, but Michael is tired, with a dry mouth. His dose is lowered to 35 mg.

WEEK 32: Michael comes in for a checkup, and his mother reports that the side effects of the Elavil have abated. The daily headaches are 50 to 70 percent improved.

THE FUTURE: The goal with children is to minimize medication yet alleviate the headaches. Because 35 mg of amitriptyline appears to be the highest dose that Michael can tolerate, if the headaches get worse, he should consider nortriptyline (Pamelor or Aventyl), a milder form of amitriptyline. While not quite as effective as amitriptyline, the nortriptyline often produces milder side effects. SSRIs (Prozac, Zoloft, Paxil) would also be considered and are usually well tolerated. A beta-blocker such as propranolol (Inderal) may help. If the headaches remain very much improved, the daily preventive medication should be discontinued periodically to assess whether it is still necessary. Many children go off and on daily preventive medication depending on the severity of their headaches. In a boy such as Michael, there is a 50 percent chance that he will outgrow the headaches by age twenty.

RICHARD

INITIAL VISIT: Richard, a seventeen-year-old high school student, has a five-year history of migraines once a month; more recently, the headaches have increased to twice a month. He also gets very mild, frequent tension headaches, but they do not bother him. The migraines are very severe, lasting sixteen to twenty-four hours, with mild nausea. All of the over-the-counter medications have been ineffective. Richard's mother and sister both have had headaches. Richard is usually a good student, but this semester he has started to stay home from school more frequently and his grades have fallen.

He and his doctor discuss diet, relaxation techniques, and the other nonmedication strategies. Richard has been using marijuana and alcohol at least three times a week. He agrees to stop, as the drugs may be responsible for worsening his headache situation. Because of his recent history of missing classes and doing poorly in school, his doctor suggests a consultation with a psychotherapist. Age seventeen is a difficult time for many adolescents, who may experience hidden stresses and depressions. Using headaches to avoid classes may also be a symptom of school phobia, which Richard needs to address with a therapist.

WEEK 4: Richard is seeing a therapist and reports that relaxation techniques have helped his milder headaches, but that the migraines persist. He receives a prescription for Midrin as an abortive medication to relieve the pain once it starts. His migraines do not occur frequently enough to justify the use of a daily preventive approach.

WEEK 6: Richard calls to say that the Midrin is mildly effective but makes him very drowsy. The doctor switches his prescription to Imitrex Nasal Spray.

WEEK 8: Richard calls to say that the Imitrex helps but he is tired from it. The doctor now prescribes Aleve, an anti-inflammatory, to be taken with Reglan, a mild antinausea medication. This is a nonaddicting, first-line medication tactic.

WEEK 20: Richard reports the medications in combination are working well.

WEEK 32: Richard reports that the Anaprox and Reglan are no longer effective. His doctor prescribes Migranal Nasal Spray. Migranal is safe, nonaddicting, and can actually abort a headache, not simply cover the pain. Richard calls after his next migraine to say it is effective.

WEEK 44: Richard phones to report that the Migranal no longer works. Richard's doctor does not want to prescribe the butalbital medications (Fiorinal, Esgic, Phrenilin) for Richard.

These drugs are mildly habit-forming, and Richard has a history of overusing alcohol and marijuana. Instead, his physician switches to another triptan, Maxalt.

WEEK 50: Richard reports that the Maxalt is working well, although he experiences twenty minutes of mild nausea after the tablet, as well as tingling in his arms. All of these side effects, however, go away easily and the headache dissipates within one hour. Richard remains slightly fatigued but is able to function well the rest of the day. He decides that he will take Maxalt with him as he goes away to college.

THE FUTURE: Other possibilities for Richard include Amerge or Zomig (other triptans), Cafergot PB suppositories, DHE injections, or, as a last resort, a butalbital compound or narcotic analgesic. Amerge may be a particularly good choice, since it is a mild, well-tolerated triptan.

12

· · · · · · · ·

HEADACHES IN PEOPLE OVER FIFTY

THE GOOD NEWS is that if you have a history of migraine, cluster, or tension headaches, chances are you'll find relief in your fifties. The bad news, though, is that many people still have problems with headaches as they get older, and some people begin getting troublesome headaches in their fifties or sixties.

If you've never had problem headaches before and are just starting to get them, or your headache patterns are suddenly changing, your doctor will probably want to do a complete workup. This is especially important as you get older. The doctor will need to be certain that the headaches are not being caused by a serious disorder that occurs more commonly as people age, such as a brain tumor, arteritis, heart disease, or high blood pressure. Other conditions that become more common as you age and that can affect headaches include depression, arthritis in the neck region, strokes from blockages in the arteries to the brain, hemorrhage in or around the brain, glaucoma or other eye conditions, or the interaction of various medications. Your doctor will also need to assess whether a cervical spine disorder, chronic renal disease, anemia, or a respiratory disorder are contributing to your headaches.

As with younger people, however, migraines, tension, and cluster headaches are also the primary headache types in people over fifty. Although headaches in older people generally are treated the same way as for younger people, some medications are not used as often. Anti-inflammatories, for example, tend to be used less often because of greater kidney and gastrointestinal problems in older people. The Cox-2 inhibitors (Celebrex, Vioxx) may be less of a problem. Triptans are used sparingly and only for people with minimal heart risk factors.

MIGRAINES AFTER AGE FIFTY

Because preventive and abortive medications for migraines are generally the same as for younger people, we will discuss only the exceptions here.

TREATING MIGRAINES IN PROGRESS

If you get a migraine, put a cold pack on the pain and rest in a dark, quiet room. If you need medication, however, your doctor will need to assess your medical conditions, such as whether you have heart risk factors, tend to experience nausea, or have the potential for addiction. Because small doses of triptans are usually used only if you have no (or minimal) heart risk factors (tell your doctor immediately if you experience any chest pains), and DHE is used increasingly sparingly for older patients, doctors tend to use the pain medications more. The anti-inflammatories, such as naproxen, are used cautiously because they tend to upset stomachs. The COX-2 inhibitors (Celebrex, Vioxx) may help. Vioxx may prove to be an outstanding medication in older age ranges.

If you don't have high blood pressure, your doctor might suggest Midrin; the doctor might also suggest low doses of one of the butalbital compounds (Fiorinal, Fioricet, Esgic, Phrenilin, Fiorinal with codeine, Fioricet with codeine), or narcotics such as hydrocodone or codeine. Occasionally, a sedative such as a benzodiazepine (such as Valium) may be helpful. If you experience nausea, tell your physician. Excedrin Migraine is an extremely effective OTC "as-needed" medication. It is usually well tolerated, but the caffeine can exacerbate insomnia and anxiety.

If you don't have any heart risk factors, Migranal (DHE) nasal spray may help by constricting blood vessels. In general, ergotamines such as Ergomar or Cafergot are not used for older people. After age seventy, mild narcotic medications are often used because of their relative safety. Phrenilin, a butalbital compound, might be useful for older people because it doesn't contain any aspirin or caffeine.

FIRST-LINE MIGRAINE PREVENTION

The first-line medications to prevent migraines are the same as described in Chapter 6 except that naproxen, an anti-inflammatory, is used less for older people. Although anti-inflammatories are generally fine for use on an "as-needed" basis, taking them on a daily basis to prevent migraines is probably not a good idea. Thus, the first-line migraine preventives are: amitriptyline (or other antidepressants), propranolol (or other beta-blockers), Depakote, and verapamil. In choosing which first-line medication is most appropriate for you, your doctor will want to assess whether anxiety, depression, insomnia, stomach problems, heartburn, inflammatory bowel syndrome, arthritis, or high blood pressure are conditions that bother you.

SECOND- AND THIRD-LINE MIGRAINE PREVENTION

If the above medications don't work, your doctor may consider combining two of them, or prescribing Neurontin. Neurontin is an excellent and safe medication that's now being widely used for pain and headaches. Methysergide (Sansert) is usually not an appropriate option if you're over fifty. If these strategies don't work or aren't appropriate for you, third-line medications include MAO inhibitors, such as phenelzine, and repetitive intravenous DHE injections. These strategies, however, are used with great caution among older people. An NSAID may also be a third-line approach. (Also see Chapter 6.)

QUICK REFERENCE GUIDE: PREVENTING
MIGRAINES AFTER AGE FIFTY

FIRST-LINE MEDICATIONS

1. AMITRIPTYLINE (OR OTHER ANTIDEPRESSANTS)

Also helps daily headaches and insomnia. SSRIs (Prozac, Zoloft, Paxil) have fewer side effects.

2. PROPRANOLOL (OR OTHER BETA-BLOCKERS)

Dosing is only once a day, but sedation, diarrhea, gastrointestinal upset, and weight gain are common.

3. VERAPAMIL

Once-a-day dosing. Nonsedating, and weight gain is uncommon, but constipation is common.

4. VALPROATE (DEPAKOTE)

Effective, but can cause fatigue or weight gain.

SECOND-LINE MEDICATIONS

1. TWO OF THE ABOVE MEDICATIONS

2. NEURONTIN

An excellent and safe medication that may cause sedation or dizziness.

THIRD-LINE MEDICATIONS

1. PHENELZINE, AN MAO INHIBITOR

Powerful and very helpful when depression, anxiety, or panic attacks are also a problem. Not appropriate if you have high blood pressure. Potentially serious side effects.

2. REPETITIVE IV DHE INJECTIONS

Used with great caution among older people. Various side effects possible. (See Chapter 6.)

3. NSAIDs

One of the last choices because of stomach upset and kidney effects. The COX-2 inhibitors (such as Vioxx) don't irritate the GI tract as much and may help.

TENSION HEADACHES AFTER AGE FIFTY

As we discussed in Chapters 8 and 9, tension headaches are common at all ages, and it's unfortunate that the name implies that tension and stress are at the root of the head pain. In fact, stress and tension may aggravate an underlying headache problem, but they are usually not the cause. The vast majority of people who get daily headaches also suffer from migraines. After age fifty, though, the migraines tend to wane, leaving a chronic daily headache.

If you are getting tension headaches less than twice a week, your doctor will probably recommend the strategies and medications discussed in Chapter 8. If you have them almost daily, you need to be careful about taking an analgesic almost every day, because doing so can make your headaches worse (see the rebound headache section in Chapter 1). If the headaches are interfering with your quality of life, however, you might ask your doctor about preventive medications.

As discussed in Chapter 9, the first-line medication used is an antidepressant, whether you're depressed or not. For older people, however, nortriptyline (Pamelor) rather than amitriplyline is generally the first medication tried because, although it's less effective, its side effects are milder. Other antidepressants, such as the SSRIs, are sometimes good choices, too. The NSAIDs are not a second choice for people over age fifty, because of the higher risk of kidney and gastrointestinal problems. With these exceptions, therapies are generally the same as those discussed in Chapter 9.

CLUSTER HEADACHES AFTER AGE FIFTY

Treatment for cluster headaches in older people is the same as that described in Chapter 10, except that fewer ergotamines (except DHE) are used. Imitrex is by far the most effective treatment. After age fifty, however, coronary artery disease (CAD), high cholesterol, diabetes, family histories of CAD, and smoking history become increasingly important with these medications. The standard older ergotamines, except for DHE, are hardly ever recommended for people over fifty. DHE, usually in the form of Migranal Nasal Spray, is sometimes useful.

In preventing cluster headaches, the discussion in Chapter 10 generally holds true for older people, with the exception of using Sansert, which is only minimally helpful for cluster headaches, and is usually not used for older people.

OTHER COMMON CAUSES OF HEADACHES IN OLDER PEOPLE

BLOCKED ARTERIES
One condition that causes headaches among people of advancing age, after migraines and tension-type headaches, is blockage of an artery that supplies blood to the brain. If the sufferer is left untreated, weakness, numbness, confusion, impaired vision, difficulty with speech, or other similar signs of dysfunction may follow. This is a serious condition and requires immediate medical attention.

HYPERTENSION
High blood pressure may cause headaches, especially in the morning. Medication should be taken to keep pressure in check. The blood pressure usually needs to be fairly high (more than 170/100) to increase headaches.

TEMPORAL ARTERITIS
This rare headache that usually afflicts only older people involves an inflammation of the temporal artery. There is a jabbing, burning pain around an ear. Other symptoms often include a low-grade fever, problems with eyesight, weight loss, and pain on one side of the jaw. Doctors still don't know the cause of these headaches, but if you experience these symptoms, see your doctor. Serious com-

plications, such as blindness, could develop if you don't. Steroids are usually the treatment of choice.

TIC DOULOUREUX (TRIGEMINAL NEURALGIA)

Also rare, these head pains are most common in women over age fifty-five. They are sharp, short, jabbing pains in the face, near the mouth or jaw. The pain, which may last from several seconds to one minute, striking many times during the day, is caused by a disease of the neural impulses. Typical treatment involves anticonvulsants, muscle relaxants, and sometimes neurosurgery or freezing of the nerve.

ARTHRITIS IN THE NECK

Arthritis may cause a low-grade, back-of-the-head ache. Physical therapy and stretching exercises may help. Anti-inflammatories may be useful, but can lead to stomach upset or ulcers. The new NSAIDs, such as Vioxx, cause less stomach bleeding or ulcers.

13
· · · · · · · ·

LESS COMMON HEADACHES
AND TREATMENTS

IN THIS CHAPTER, we'll look at other kinds of headaches that
are actually less common, though some are very well known, such
as sinus headaches and sexual headaches. In most cases, these
headaches are named for their triggers and are similar to the types
of headaches we have discussed so far. Nevertheless, many people
identify their headache by its triggers, so it's useful to address each
one separately.

POST-TRAUMATIC HEADACHE

Headaches are very common after a rear-end car accident,
whether or not your head or neck was injured in the collision.
This is particularly true if you have suffered from headaches before. Usually these headaches develop within hours or days of the
accident, although occasionally they may begin months later. In
most cases, the headaches will taper off within a few days to several weeks. However, even minor accidents can produce very severe, long-lasting headaches of up to a year or more.

Post-traumatic headaches are usually either tension-type
headaches — daily or episodic — or more severe migraine-type
headaches, or both. Neck and back-of-the-head pain are also very
common. The pain comes from damage to muscles, ligaments, and
occasionally to intervertebral discs. Tenderness or stiffness and
pain in the neck and shoulder muscles are quite common. This
pain may be resistant to therapy, but physical therapy or chiro-

practic manipulations may be helpful. Typical symptoms that may accompany these headaches are poor concentration, becoming easily angered or frustrated, sensitivity to noise or bright lights, depression, dizziness, ringing in the ears, memory problems, fatigue, insomnia, lack of motivation, lessening sexual drive, nervousness or anxiety, irritability, and decreased ability to comprehend complex issues.

It is difficult to predict who will continue to suffer chronic, unremitting post-traumatic pain after an accident. If you were in a rear-end collision but didn't injure your head, you might still get severe headaches and neck pain. The angle of impact, where you were sitting in the car, and what happened to your brain within the skull are key elements in whether you'll get headaches afterward.

The older you are, the more likely you are to develop post-traumatic headaches after an accident. Women are almost twice as likely to suffer from post-traumatic headaches as men. If you tended to get headaches or had migraine problems before the accident, or have a very strong family history of headaches, you also are at higher risk. Although the severity of your accident or injury might predict your likelihood of suffering post-traumatic headache, many people endure months or years of severe post-traumatic headaches after even very trivial collisions. Studies disagree as to whether many of these people exaggerate or malinger, although researchers have noted that even after other issues are settled (litigation, disability, worker's compensation, insurance), most people continue having the same degree of symptoms, suggesting that few people actually fake their pain.

Nevertheless, many people with post-traumatic headaches often do not receive much sympathy from physicians, coworkers, friends, or family members, with the result that the situation can spiral into a vicious cycle of psychological stress. You may already feel disabled because of frequent headaches after an accident and then feel the additional stress of difficulty at home or work due to your headaches, anxiety, insomnia, and attention or concentration difficulties. Most people at this point admit that they don't care much about the insurance, litigation, or worker's compensation, saying, "All I want to do is get back to normal." To make matters worse, objective testing does not reveal problems in the vast majority of these injured people, and they are often not fairly compensated by legal and insurance processes. Although most people with post-traumatic headaches improve within weeks, a small but important percentage of them continue to suffer for months, years, or a lifetime.

If you've been in an accident or endured some other kind of head injury that is now causing headaches (or some of the other symptoms we've listed), you should definitely consult a doctor to assess the physical injury. The doctor may suggest physical therapy, psychological counseling, relaxation training or biofeedback, medication, or a combination of these treatments.

RELIEVING POST-TRAUMATIC HEADACHES WITH MEDICATION

In the first few weeks of headaches, anti-inflammatories (aspirin, ibuprofen, and naproxen) are usually recommended because they not only help with the head pain but can also help relieve any accompanying neck or back pain. If these drugs are ineffective, the doctor may next recommend a choice from the list of medications used for tension headaches and migraines, depending on which type the pain most closely resembles. Muscle relaxants like cyclobenzaprine (Flexeril) or methocarbamol (Robaxin) may also be helpful if spasms occur in the neck, but these medications may cause fatigue.

Most people with post-traumatic migraines need only abortive medications because the headaches resolve themselves over time. However, if the headaches are migraines, occur frequently, or cause you to use excessive amounts of abortive medication, a preventive strategy may be recommended.

The antidepressants, particularly amitriptyline (Elavil) or nortriptyline (Pamelor), Depakote, and the beta-blockers (Inderal, Corgard) are the most commonly prescribed preventives used for post-traumatic headaches. The sedating antidepressants, particularly amitriptyline, often help relieve daily headaches, migraines, and any associated insomnia. In severe cases, a combination of these may be recommended. The anti-inflammatories may also be used as a preventive.

If the headaches are migraines, your doctor may recommend calcium blockers (verapamil) as a first-line therapy. SSRIs (Prozac, Paxil, Zoloft, Celexa) may help, particularly if you also have anxiety or depression or both. Intravenous DHE, given repetitively in the office or in the hospital, is very useful with severe cases and is used along with a daily preventive medication. "As-needed" medications need to be limited, following the steps outlined in previous chapters. The triptans (Imitrex, Amerge, Maxalt, Zomig, Relpax) are particularly useful for migraines.

EXERCISE AND SEXUAL HEADACHES

Exertional headaches are divided into three main categories:

1. Benign exertional headache
2. Headache associated with sexual activity
3. Benign cough headache

If physical exercise triggers headaches, and serious problems, such as brain tumors, have been excluded, then you are experiencing benign exertional headaches. Typically, this type of headache is felt on both sides of the head and usually throbs, occasionally occurring with nausea. These headaches usually last from minutes to twenty-four hours, and are not linked with serious problems, such as brain tumors. Hot weather and high altitude may make these exertional headaches more likely to occur. Keeping well hydrated can help. "Smoother" exercises such as walking and biking are less likely to trigger exertional headaches.

If you've never had exertional headaches and you suddenly get them, you should call your doctor or go to the emergency room immediately. As with all headaches, new-onset exertional headaches are more worrisome than those of long-standing origin. Headaches that begin extremely explosively and rise to a crescendo within one minute are particularly potentially serious. Your doctor will need to first check that you have no serious problems in the brain that are causing them, such as a brain tumor, an aneurysm that can cause bleeding, or other similar problems. Your doctor may need to do an MRI (magnetic resonance imaging), MRA, plain x-ray of the skull, blood tests, or even a lumbar puncture (spinal tap) to rule out more severe causes. Fortunately, however, the vast majority of these exertional headaches are benign and are not associated with serious problems in the brain.

Headaches that come on with sexual activity usually begin on both sides of the head; often, stopping the sexual activity immediately can halt the headache. One type of sexual headache causes a dull ache about the head or neck that increases as sexual excitement escalates. A second more explosive type is very severe and occurs with orgasm. Benign cough headache is usually very sudden, lasting less than one minute, and is on both sides of the head.

Typically, benign exertional headaches occur in people who are in their twenties and thirties, sexual headache occurs more in middle age (at approximately age forty), and a cough headache typically comes in the sixties. More men than women have these exertional headaches.

Obviously, to prevent exertional headaches, you can avoid the exercise or the sex that tends to trigger them, though many people are not willing or able to do this. The usual preventive treatment is an anti-inflammatory medication, such as indomethacin (Indocin) or naproxen (Aleve). Ibuprofen (Motrin) or flurbiprofen (Ansaid) may also be effective. These medications are usually given one half to two hours prior to the activity. The effective dose varies widely, but the usual doses are: indomethacin, 50 mg to 75 mg; Aleve, two tablets; ibuprofen, 600 mg; flurbiprofen, one or two of the 100-mg tablets. While triptans may be effective, doctors do not usually encourage the taking of a triptan (Imitrex, Maxalt, Amerge, Zomig) prior to exercise.

If you get an exertional headache, apply ice to your head, lie down in a dark room, and take one of the medications described for migraine and tension headaches. (For a discussion of these "as-needed" migraine or tension headache medications, see Chapters 5 and 8.)

SPINAL TAP HEADACHES

About one-third of people who have spinal taps, a diagnostic procedure, get lumbar puncture headaches. Although anyone can get one, women with a history of headaches and younger, underweight people are at highest risk.

The smaller the needle used, the smaller the risk of a subsequent headache. The position you assume after the procedure, the experience of the doctor, or the amount of spinal fluid taken do *not* appear to affect the likelihood of getting such a headache. Psychological factors play a lesser role than was once thought.

Usually the headache comes on within forty-eight hours of the spinal tap, but occasionally it may not occur until two weeks afterward. The pain may be in the front or back of the head, or in the neck and shoulder area. Typically, it hurts to sit or stand, but lying down can help. The pain may be throbbing, pounding, or ache severely.

The symptoms resemble those of migraines — nausea, visual disturbances, sensitivity to light, and dizziness — but in addition, neck pain and spasm often occur. Usually the headaches resolve themselves within days to weeks, occasionally longer. Just what causes the headaches is not known for sure, though some experts believe the mechanism may be similar to that of migraines.

For most people, simply using analgesics, as described in Chapter 2, is all that's necessary until the headaches decline. Although oral caffeine may help, it's hard to consume enough to make a significant difference. If the headache persists for more than two days, your doctor may recommend an injection of caffeine. Be warned, however, that it can cause central nervous system side effects such as jitters or tremors, as well as a rapid heartbeat. Drinking at least six glasses of liquid each day may also help.

If the headache is severe and unimproving, an epidural blood patch — an injection of your own blood in the lower back, where the spinal tap was done — can be extremely effective. This is an easy procedure for an experienced physician. And if this treatment doesn't work, then standard tension headache prevention medications may be recommended, as well as a saline solution injection near the spinal tap puncture.

SINUS HEADACHES

Although many people think they suffer from chronic sinus headaches, chances are they are experiencing mild migraines. Very few chronic headaches — less than 2 percent of all headaches and less than 30 percent of recurring headaches believed to be sinus headaches — actually fit into this category.

It can be exceedingly difficult to determine the cause of a frontal, or facial, headache associated with nasal congestion or stuffiness. In certain seasons or during weather changes, many people with migraines do experience a stuffy frontal headache, which they mistake for a sinus headache. A combined approach, treating both the migraines and nasal congestion, may be necessary.

Most sinus headaches are caused by infections and fluid buildup in the bony pockets of the upper face. This congestion causes pressure and pain and usually a fever. Symptoms include a runny or stuffy nose, postnasal drip, and tenderness around the sinus regions of the face. X-rays can confirm the diagnosis of sinusitis, though a CAT scan is the best tool for looking at this area. An MRI of the brain also lets doctors "see" the area. Antibiotics are often needed to treat the infection.

Migraines, on the other hand, are far more common than true sinus headaches but are often misidentified because they also can cause pain in the sinuses. Migraine pain is caused by the dilation of blood vessels — which may occur in the face and sinus region — as well as by irritated nerves that misfire the pain signal along the head's large trigeminal nerve, with branches throughout the face and sinus. Thus, pain in the sinus region may have nothing to do with the sinuses.

If you think you have a sinus headache and decide to take an over-the-counter sinus medication, it may work because it contains caffeine, an analgesic (aspirin or acetaminophen), or a vasoconstrictor — all substances that would help a migraine. Sinus medications with decongestants, however, can make your headache worse if it is not a true sinus headache because they can raise your blood pressure and aggravate the source of your pain. Do not overuse the OTC nasal sprays. Prescription cortisone-based nasal sprays are more effective and do not produce rebound nasal stuffiness. Many people suffer from both migraine and sinus headaches and distinguishing between the two can be a challenge.

ALLERGY HEADACHES

Although allergies and headaches are both very common, allergies usually do not cause headaches. When you experience an allergy attack, you may get a headache, however, because your nasal and sinus blood vessels are more sensitive. When smoke, chocolate, or red wine, for example, cause a headache, it's probably not because you are allergic to them but because you are sensitive to their effect on blood vessels. Much more commonly, these headaches are a migraine- or a tension-type headache. A true allergy headache, caused by an immune system that misfires, occurs only occasionally and is triggered by pollen, molds, and other common allergens. Its symptoms are very similar to hay fever: a runny nose, sneezing, watery eyes, and sometimes a sore throat, with pain usually in the front, above and below the eyes.

Of course there are food allergies, but they more typically cause nausea, vomiting, hives, wheezing, diarrhea, rashes, and itching rather than headaches. Allergies to dairy foods and wheat products (bread and pasta) are the most common. Keep a headache diary and try to distinguish between a food sensitivity and an allergy; in either case, if you can identify the food that is triggering your headaches, avoid it. Prescription nasal (cortisone-based) sprays and antihistamines occasionally help frontal headaches.

However, allergy treatments usually help the allergies themselves much more than they help the related migraines.

TEMPOROMANDIBULAR JOINT (TMJ) HEADACHES, JAW CLENCHING, AND BRUXISM

While disorders of the jaw and teeth are generally overdiagnosed as a cause of headache, TMJ problems, clenching, and bruxism may *add* to a headache patient's pain. (Bruxism is not only clenching but also grinding the teeth from side to side.) It can be very difficult, however, to assess accurately the extent to which someone's teeth clenching or TMJ problem is adding to a headache situation.

Some headaches are related to problems with the temporomandibular joint, the hinge attaching the lower jaw to the skull. It is located just in front of each ear, and if you move your jaw you can feel it. When this area is sensitive to touch, especially with a dull or stabbing headache, the headache may be related to a disorder of the joint but may also be a migraine or tension headache. If you have trouble opening or closing your jaw all the way, if your jaw locks, or you are sore in the jaw muscles TMJ may be the problem. Usually these headaches can be relieved with the same strategies used for tension headaches (see Chapters 2 and 8). Check with a doctor or dentist if they persist. Some people clench their teeth and jaw all day or at night, leading to increased headaches. A dentist or TMJ specialist can give you a mouth bite splint to stop you from clenching. Many people suffer from clenching and bruxism *plus* tension or migraine headaches.

EYESTRAIN HEADACHES

When we overuse our eyes or do not have the proper corrective lenses, we overwork the muscles around our eyes, which can cause a tension headache. A headache from eyestrain is usually a dull, frontal ache or pain behind the eyes.

Of course, the same medications that help tension headaches will relieve eyestrain headaches, but an eye exam and improved corrective lenses would probably go further in preventing them in the future! Contact lenses do not usually offer an advantage over glasses in regard to headache. Computer screens may exacerbate eyestrain. Taking frequent breaks and using an anti-glare screen may help.

HANGOVER HEADACHES

Alcohol can cause throbbing headaches (with or without nausea) by dilating and irritating blood vessels, wreaking havoc on the blood sugar–insulin balance, causing dehydration, or introducing chemicals to which the body is sensitive. The most effective way to treat a hangover headache is to drink as much water as possible as well as some fruit juice or to eat some honey on crackers and take two aspirin. These strategies are most effective if taken before bed and upon awakening. People who experience migraines may be more susceptible to hangover headaches.

"ICE CREAM" HEADACHES

Some people are particularly sensitive to very cold foods, such as ice cream, and coldness may trigger sudden and severe pain in the forehead, nose, temples, or cheeks. The pain usually lasts less than a minute. It helps to eat the cold food slowly. These headaches are caused because of stimulating a nerve in the back of the throat.

TIGHT-HAT HEADACHES

As most people know, a tight hat, swimming cap, headband, or swimming goggles may cause pressure or irritate the nerves around the head and trigger a headache. In the vast majority of cases, these headaches can be simply treated with the over-the-counter analgesics described in Chapter 2. People who get tension or migraine headaches are particularly susceptible.

WEEKEND AND TRAVEL HEADACHES

If you drink a lot of coffee and tea at work and don't continue this pattern on the weekend, you may get weekend headaches, which are very common. So-called caffeine withdrawal usually occurs some eighteen to thirty-six hours after the last cup of coffee or tea. Travel can wreak the same kind of havoc on your normal caffeine consumption.

These headaches can be decreased by gradually diminishing the amount of caffeine you regularly ingest so your body is not so dependent on it. Or you can be more careful in maintaining a constant level of caffeine consumption on weekends or trips. Going to bed and awakening at the same time as on the weekday may also help.

If you get headaches after a stressful week and get a so-called Saturday morning migraine, you may need to remember to incorporate stress-reducing techniques in your week, such as physical exercise or relaxation exercises to relieve the build-up of stress and how your body holds it. These weekend stress-letdown headaches are often exceedingly difficult to treat and eliminate. It may help to remain busy on weekends, rather than going from a period of high activity to doing nothing. At times, preventive medication may be used on Friday and Saturday only (for example, taking two Aleve on Friday night and Saturday morning).

HOLIDAY HEADACHES

Some people complain that their headaches flare up during the holiday season. A combination of factors, such as the stress and frustration of getting all their holiday shopping and chores done in time, fighting crowds and traffic, and the extra strain of attending numerous social events with coworkers or relatives, is probably responsible. Also, people tend to drink more alcohol and disrupt their routines during the holidays, which can contribute to triggering headaches. Headache sufferers are particularly susceptible to disruptions in their sleeping and eating schedules. The strategies in Chapter 2 (relaxation and stress-reduction exercises and perhaps an over-the-counter pain reliever) will help keep the holidays headache-free.

AFTER-SURGERY HEADACHES

Doctors have noticed for years that patients often experience headaches after surgery. Recent studies suggest that these are actually caffeine-withdrawal headaches because of the requirement that you not eat or drink anything twelve hours prior to the surgery. Discuss this possibility with your doctor prior to surgery.

After surgery, eating and having a cup of tea or coffee and a mild over-the-counter painkiller (aspirin, acetaminophen, or ibuprofen) will probably relieve these headaches. In any case, they resolve themselves quickly.

There is anecdotal evidence that some people actually experience a *decrease* in migraines for several months after surgery. The reason for this is not known.

HEMICRANIA CONTINUA

Hemicrania continua are rare one-sided headaches of dull, throbbing pain. Severe pain may occur, lasting from five to sixty minutes, three to five times per twenty-four hours. The pain is usually pulsating, with several minutes of intensely painful ice-pick jabs. Men and women of all ages suffer equally. Alcohol or physical exertion often intensifies the pain. Some people may experience other symptoms similar to migraines, such as sensitivity to light and nausea.

The anti-inflammatory indomethacin is the drug of choice for hemicrania continua headaches and will relieve them in 80 percent of cases. If you can't tolerate it, or if it isn't helpful, then your doctor will probably follow the strategies for migraine prevention, suggesting amitriptyline, naproxen, or calcium blockers.

CHRONIC PAROXYSMAL HEMICRANIA (CPH)

These very rare chronic cluster headaches are treated differently from other clusters. Most common among young women between twenty-five and thirty-five, these headaches are usually one-sided and focused around an eye, temple, or the forehead. Typically, the pain lasts up to fifteen minutes and may strike anywhere from five to twenty times a day. Like other types of cluster headaches, the pain is extremely severe and often associated with a tearing eye and a stuffy or runny nose.

Such severe headaches should be assessed by a doctor to exclude the rare possibility of a tumor or an aneurysm. Once diagnosed properly, CPH headaches are almost always relieved by the anti-inflammatory indomethacin (Indocin), though the effective dose varies greatly, from as little as 25 mg to 250 mg per day. The medication should always be taken with food to avoid gastrointestinal upset. Other side effects of the medication include fatigue, light-headedness, and mood swings. Liver and kidney blood tests need to be checked regularly to rule out any organ dysfunction.

BACK-OF-THE-HEAD SHARP PAIN
(OCCIPITAL NEURALGIA)

About 20 percent of migraine sufferers, as well as other headache sufferers, sometimes experience a sharp, burning, ice-pick or stabbing pain in the back of the head (occipital neuralgia). It may be accompanied by tenderness around the nerve in that area.

If severe, the pain can be relieved with a nerve-block injection of an anesthetic (Marcaine or lidocaine) just under the skin. The procedure is easy, with minimal discomfort and low risk. The injection may be done once or twice but usually not more than several times a year. If effective, the pain may be relieved for weeks or months. These so-called occipital nerve blockades are also helpful for cluster headaches and their variants, such as chronic paroxysmal hemicrania. Cortisone injections in the area of the nerve are sometimes more effective.

Back-of-the-head pain may also stem from injury, such as whiplash, or from shingles (herpes zoster). While antidepressants, anti-inflammatories, or the anticonvulsants carbamazepine (Tegretol) or gabapentin (Neurontin) relieve such pain, many people with occipital neuralgia respond better to injections. Physical therapy to the neck occasionally is helpful.

NECK PROBLEMS CAUSING HEADACHE (CERVICOGENIC HEADACHE)

It's controversial whether neck headache (cervicogenic headache) is a distinct type of headache or is a type of migraine or tension headache. These headaches consist of one-sided back-of-the-head pain, usually accompanied by tension in the neck muscles and muscle spasm. Moving the neck often brings on the pain. Symptoms of migraines may also occur, such as blurred vision or nausea. Other symptoms may include arm pain, tearing of the eye, difficulty swallowing, numbness, and ringing of the ears. An MRI (magnetic resonance imaging) of the neck and other tests usually do not reveal problems. A doctor will probably treat these headaches as migraine or tension headaches. Injections of Novocain or cortisone (trigger-point injections) in the back of the head area or the back of the neck area may also be helpful.

MEDICATION-INDUCED HEADACHES

Almost all medication labels list headache as a possible side effect. Even patients who take a placebo sometimes report headaches.

The *Physicians' Desk Reference* and other medication reference books often list headaches as a side effect or adverse reaction to many medications.

In susceptible individuals, almost any medication may bring on a headache, even acetaminophen, aspirin, or ibuprofen. A few medications, however, that are commonly linked to headaches include atenolol, captropril, cimetidine, cocaine, danazol, diclofenac, nitroglycerin, hormones (estrogen or progesterone), oral contraceptives, and ranitidine (Zantac). In addition, calcium blockers, such as verapamil, can produce a chronic daily low-grade headache, and antidepressants, such as amitriptyline or SSRIs, can increase the frequency of headaches in some people. Ironically, these medications are often prescribed for headaches because they help decrease headaches in more than half of patients who take them and aggravate headaches in only about 5 percent. Likewise, anti-inflammatories, such as ibuprofen, aspirin, and naproxen, also prescribed for headaches, occasionally aggravate a headache situation.

As we've mentioned in previous chapters, many analgesics produce rebound headaches when patients overuse them, especially medications with caffeine, which include many of the over-the-counter pain relievers. Although caffeine helps headaches when taken in small amounts, too much caffeine on a daily basis may increase headaches. Ergotamine preparations, which temporarily shrink the arteries, also often produce rebound headaches in daily dosers.

Many medications used to protect the heart or to lower blood pressure will help headaches while others induce more headaches. Nitroglycerin, for example, a medication prescribed for heart problems, often produces a headache. Antibiotics and cold preparations may also bring on headaches in some people.

Fact: Almost any medication can increase headaches in a susceptible individual.

HEADACHES CAUSED BY MEDICAL CONDITIONS

Many other factors can cause headaches, such as too much sun, high blood pressure, and a host of medical disorders.

INFECTIONS

In a headache-prone person, any infection may induce headaches. A migraine sufferer with a sinus infection or the flu will probably experience a more severe and prolonged headache than a nonmigraine sufferer. Yet infections can also induce moderate to severe headaches in people who have never had a migraine or tension headache.

Headaches are also common with fevers, which are an indication of an infection. Fevers tend to bring on general head pain that's caused by the blood vessels in the head expanding. Treatment involves aspirin, acetaminophen, and antibiotics.

Meningitis (an infection involving the covering of the brain) usually produces a fever, headache, and stiff neck. HIV headache can cause severe pain, is often related to light sensitivity, and almost always occurs in conjunction with advanced infection. Any headache associated with a fever should be reported to a physician. While people with HIV may experience headaches for a number of reasons, pre-existing migraines may actually diminish with the onset of AIDS.

CIRCULATORY PROBLEMS

Although most migraine sufferers experience cold feet or hands, true circulatory problems do not occur more often in headache patients than among the general population.

Stroke may produce headaches in some people, but the pain is usually minimal. Heart disease and artery disease in the arms or legs (peripheral vascular disease) do not usually cause headaches, although medications used to treat these conditions occasionally exacerbate or induce a headache.

HIGH BLOOD PRESSURE

Uncontrolled high blood pressure on a moderate to severe level may cause or exacerbate headaches. Usually, these headaches are felt around the head or at the "hatband." They tend to be worse in the morning and get better as the day goes on. They occur in people with severe hypertension, with over 180 systolic and 110 diastolic pressure. Treatment involves medication to keep the blood pressure in check. *Mild* elevations in blood pressure, however, do *not* usually increase the severity or frequency of headaches. On the other hand, during the day of a migraine or cluster headache, many people will experience a rise in blood pressure.

CANCER

Brain tumors may cause or aggravate headaches, but cancer in other parts of the body usually does not significantly affect head pain. Brain tumors are rare and usually coupled with progressively worse vomiting and increased head pain upon coughing and sneezing. Cancer patients should report any new neurologic symptom, such as vision changes or numbness, to a doctor. Certain medications used to treat cancer or associated medical complications may increase headaches in some people.

EYE PROBLEMS

Although some severe eye problems, such as glaucoma, can cause eye pain or headache, such pain usually does not involve the eyes themselves. Nevertheless, an exam with an ophthalmologist may be very helpful to rule out the eyes as a contributing factor in headache. (Eyestrain was discussed earlier in this chapter.)

EAR PROBLEMS

Pain in or about the ear may represent ear disease or referred pain from the jaw joint, as in TMJ, which was discussed earlier in this chapter. Migraine sufferers occasionally experience a sharp, stabbing pain in or around the ear. However, migraine pain is rarely limited to the ear. When the pain around an ear is steady and constant, it is probably caused by an inner ear infection and needs a doctor's attention.

HYPOGLYCEMIA

Most physicians do not believe that hypoglycemia is a real factor in headaches. However, *normal* drops in blood sugar (not *true* hypoglycemia) can produce a "hunger" headache (though not necessarily a migraine) in some migraine sufferers, particularly if they haven't eaten for twelve or more hours. Diabetics who experience low blood sugar or whose diabetes is not well controlled may also get a headache, even a migraine. A glass of orange juice or a sugary food should relieve the low blood sugar and the head pain.

MISCELLANEOUS FACTORS

Some environmental contaminants may also contribute to headaches. These include air pollution, benzene, carbon monoxide, formaldehyde, glutaraldehyde, hydrogen sulfide, methyl alcohol, toluene, trichloroethylene, and xylene. Other activities that may induce headaches include jet lag, an epileptic seizure, and lactation.

14

· · · · · · · · ·

MORE ALTERNATIVES

THE TECHNIQUES in this chapter, some of them unorthodox, can be very effective. Whether these strategies provide relief directly or offer a placebo is not known. The placebo effect is real and powerful — some 35 percent of headache sufferers report short-term relief after taking a pill that they expect to work. However, the placebo effect usually diminishes in the course of one to two months.

Although we do not necessarily prescribe or recommend any of these treatments, we do think it is important to let you know about the many options available. When appropriate, discuss them with your physician. The most prominent alternative treatments are herbs, aromatherapy, physical therapy, trigger-point injections, massage, and vitamins and minerals.

HERBS

You might benefit from one or several herbs. One problem with herbs, however, is that there is little quality control and standardization. Because of differences in species, soil, weather conditions, and additives, different preparations of herbs (with the same milligram strength) may have widely varying strength and purities. One recent study of ten different preparations of St.-John's-Wort and feverfew, for example, revealed extreme differences among herbs from different farms in the strength of the active ingredient in each capsule.

Despite these drawbacks, herbs have a wide appeal because of their general safety and less severe side effects. But virtually everything has possible side effects, and many of these herbs can interact with other drugs and various medical conditions. Tell your doctor exactly what herbs you are taking, as there can be significant interactions.

Feverfew is the primary herb used to prevent migraine. Ginger can help fight nausea, especially migraine nausea. Valerian is used as a natural tranquilizer and sleep aid, which helps some headaches. Chamomile or kava kava may be useful as a mild sedative. There is now a *Physicians' Desk Reference* for herbs available in the United States, as well as several excellent books, including *Herbs of Choice* by Varro E. Tyler, Ph.D., Sc.D. (Pharmaceutical Products Press).

FEVERFEW *(Tanacetum parthenium)*

Feverfew has been used to bring fevers down since at least the first century A.D., and its use in headache dates to the early 1600s. Feverfew is a wildflower in the chrysanthemum family that is very easy to grow in backyards. This herb has been shown to be mildly effective in reducing the frequency and severity of migraine headaches in a number of reasonably controlled studies. The active ingredient appears to be parthenolide — a compound that inhibits or decreases the clumping up of platelets in the bloodstream and may affect prostaglandins. The result of parthenolide activity may be a decreased release of serotonin in the bloodstream. Serotonin is, as we have seen, a key in headaches. While many people chew the leaves of feverfew, it is easier (but possibly not more effective) to obtain the standardized capsules or tablets.

The usual dose is 125 mg of dried feverfew, containing at least 0.2 percent parthenolide, once per day. The standardized extract is also available in 200-mg doses, containing up to 0.7 percent parthenolide. Liquid extract and whole-herb capsules are also available. Doctors usually advise two capsules or tablets per day, because one may not have the potency that is necessary. An adequate daily dose of parthenolide is 250 mcg. While this amount should be contained in the 125-mg capsule or tablet, taking two would usually ensure at least the minimum necessary to help headaches.

Unfortunately, feverfew may take as long as six or eight weeks to become effective. Occasionally, capsules of feverfew or feverfew with caffeine or feverfew with guarana (which is essentially caffeine) are used either as a preventive or to treat a headache in progress. These are available from Eclectic Farms, (800) 332-4372. The usual dose would be two or three capsules or tablets. Taking caffeine with the feverfew may increase the effectiveness.

Feverfew should not be used during pregnancy or by women who are nursing. Side effects include minor mouth ulcerations in 10 to 12 percent of people, irritation of the tongue or the mouth in 7 to 12 percent, stomach upset, and possibly an increased tendency toward bleeding. Do not take feverfew if you are on a blood thinner, such as Coumadin. If you take aspirin, it is theoretically possible that feverfew could increase your bleeding time. People occasionally demonstrate an allergy to the feverfew. This may be more likely if you are allergic to plants of the ragweed family.

GINGER

Ginger, in capsule form, is used to offset nausea. One or two capsules every four hours, as needed, four per day at most, is the standard dose. The whole herb capsules are usually 500 mg, and the standardized dried extract is often available in 150-mg doses. An increased tendency toward bleeding or prolonging of bleeding is one possible side effect. Ginger can be used to fight motion sickness, too.

VALERIAN

Valerian is probably the most effective herbal tranquilizer and sleep aid. It's relatively safe, with few side effects. The usual dose is one or two capsules every day as needed, or one teaspoon in one cup of water (prepared as tea). At high doses, headache may ensue. It has been recommended that valerian not be used daily for long periods of time, but long-term toxicity is unlikely.

CHAMOMILE

Chamomile is a mild sedative or relaxant and antinausea herb; it may also be useful for other digestive problems, since it is a mild antispasmodic (it relaxes the smooth muscle of the digestive tract). There are a number of forms of chamomile, primarily the German versus the English (Roman) varieties. In the United States, German chamomile is most commonly available. As with most herbs, there may be differences in effectiveness among the various species. Chamomile is felt to be a very safe herb. Since chamomile is relatively expensive and easy to adulterate, quality control has been a problem. Previous studies on commercial chamomile oil have indicated a high rate of adulteration. The whole-herb capsules are often available in 355-mg doses, and liquid extract or tea bags are also available.

ST.-JOHN'S-WORT *(Hypericum perforatum)*

St.-John's-Wort is a very popular herbal remedy for mild depression and may also be useful for anxiety. It may work by activity on the monoamine oxidase (MAO) system. St.-John's-Wort may take four to eight weeks to become effective for depression. For more than very mild depression, the antidepressants or psychotherapy have generally been more useful. Side effects have included stomach complaints, and in rare cases, when someone is taking large doses, skin photosensitivity (increased sensitivity to sunlight). St.-John's-Wort should not be used concurrently with other antidepressants. Most 300-mg capsules contain from 0.15 percent hypericin to 0.3 percent hypericin. You should be under a doctor's supervision if you are using St.-John's-Wort for depression. The optimum dose is not known.

KAVA KAVA *(Piper methysticum)*

Kava kava is an anti-anxiety herb that may also be useful for mild insomnia. It is not recommended for those with serious depression, as it possibly has the potential to increase suicide risk. Kava should also not be used during pregnancy or if you are nursing. Rarely, allergic reactions or yellowing of the skin have been reported. Stomach upset also may occur. Kava may increase the sedative effect of alcohol or other sedative drugs. The daily dose has been approximately equivalent to 60 mg to 120 mg of kava pyrones. Kava is often available as a whole-herb extract (300 mg) or a standardized extract capsule of 250 mg (which contains 30 percent kava lactones, or about 75 mg kava lactones).

GINGKO BILOBA

Gingko has not demonstrated any clear efficacy in headache. It is most likely better utilized for memory disturbances, circulation problems, or possibly to counteract the sexual side effects of antidepressants.

WILLOW BARK

Willow bark (white willow bark is commonly used) contains salicin, an aspirinlike compound that inhibits prostaglandins. While safe in recommended doses, this compound is probably not very effective because it is too difficult to achieve the sufficient doses that are necessary.

GUARANA

Guarana contains caffeine in its seeds. It is usually used in the form of crushed (powdered) seeds. It is effective for headache primarily because of its high caffeine content. There are no major advantages in using guarana over caffeine.

PEPPERMINT

Peppermint has occasionally been used to help certain digestive problems; it might be helpful for calming an upset stomach associated with migraine. Peppermint is available as leaves, capsules, liquid extract, or oil extracts.

VITAMINS AND MINERALS

Several vitamins and minerals have been found to be useful to prevent headaches. In studies, magnesium is proving to be the most successful one, but vitamin B_2 (riboflavin), vitamin B_6 (pyridoxine), vitamin B_{12} (cyanocobalamin), calcium, and certain long-chain fatty acids that are contained in compounds such as fish oil or flaxseed oil might also be useful.

MAGNESIUM

A number of studies have shown that the brains of migraine sufferers have low levels of magnesium, which is important for arteries and serotonin to function. When magnesium levels are too low, arteries tend to constrict or become more narrow. That's why magnesium infusions help severe migraines. However, taking magnesium daily supplements to prevent or decrease headaches, especially menstrual migraines, is the most popular use. Dark green leafy vegetables, whole-grain breads or cereals, seafood, legumes, and nuts are all high in magnesium. (However, certain legumes, such as lima, navy, fava, garbanzo, pinto, and Italian beans and lentils, trigger migraines in some people, as do nuts.)

If you want to try magnesium as a supplement, 250-mg doses once or twice per day are common and deemed safe. Try to avoid magnesium sulfate; take magnesium oxide instead. Some of the supplements can cause diarrhea, but magnesium oxide usually does not. It is possible that the slow-release or chelated form of magnesium has advantages over the regular magnesium supplements, primarily because of improved absorption. People with kidney problems, however, should avoid magnesium supplements.

After several months, it might be a good idea to stop taking magnesium, as long-term side effects have not been firmly established.

VITAMIN B₂ (RIBOFLAVIN)

Several studies have shown that large doses of this B vitamin (400 mg per day) are more effective in preventing migraine headaches than a placebo. In one fairly small study, for example, those who took 400 mg daily for several months experienced almost 40 percent fewer migraines: these results need to be interpreted with some caution. Also, it took at least a month for any clinical effect. Doctors do not usually use this treatment for more than six months, as long-term toxic side effects of large doses of vitamin B_2 have not been established. However, in general, the B vitamins are safe.

CALCIUM

Calcium has been reported in at least one study to decrease premenstrual symptoms and menstrual headaches. If you take calcium and magnesium, take them at different times of the day, as the calcium may inhibit the absorption of magnesium. Food sources of calcium include dark green leafy vegetables, dairy products, seafood, and certain fish. Supplements are usually necessary, 750 mg to 1,500 mg per day.

VITAMIN B₆ (PYRIDOXINE) AND B₁₂ (CYANOCOBALAMIN)

Vitamin B_6 is used to prevent migraines, particularly menstrual migraines. Typical and safe doses are 50 mg or 100 mg per day. Many people have found that taking a B complex (B-100) helps their headaches. It is known that the B vitamins, particularly folate and B_{12}, can help prevent heart disease and possibly stroke. Recent studies indicate that B_{12} (which is poorly absorbed orally) may be helpful in preventing headaches.

LONG-CHAIN FATTY ACIDS (PRIMARILY OMEGA-3 AND OMEGA-6 FATTY ACIDS)

Certain types of fatty acids that are present in fish oil concentrate and flaxseed oil may help headache. These have also been demonstrated to be useful in certain types of anxiety or mood disorders. Because of the problems with fish oil, doctors usually recommend flaxseed oil, 1,000-mg capsules, one or two per day. This is a fairly low dose; much higher doses have been used. These fatty acids may be beneficial for prevention of heart disease as well.

AROMATHERAPY

Aromatherapy may work when small molecules of essential oils become absorbed into the skin or respiratory tract and directly stimulate the smell sense nerve (olfactory nerve). This nerve is widely distributed with connections throughout the brain. Aromatherapy may be useful for milder headaches, such as the usual tension headaches. Some people can take less medication when they use aromatherapy. A recent study revealed peppermint oil to be as useful as aspirin for pure tension headaches.

The oils should be stored in dark glass bottles; buy the ones with the words "distilled" and "pure" on them. Keep them out of sunlight and intense heat. These essential oils should not be used orally but rather inhaled or applied to the temples, neck, or shoulder muscles. Since the essential oils are very potent, use only very small amounts. For instance, one drop of the oil is usually diluted in a teaspoon of almond oil (or another carrier oil) and then rubbed into the skin. Alternatively, four to seven drops of the oil may be put into warm water for a bath.

The most commonly utilized oils for headache are peppermint, lavender, and chamomile. The Roman chamomile (English chamomile) has been used in aromatherapy more than the German chamomile. Lavender and peppermint may be the most useful in this group. In addition to these, tiger balm is a powerful herb that has been used extensively in China. Eucalyptus has been a popular aromatherapy for sinus-type headaches.

If aromatherapy is used for migraine, beware that intense smells may increase nausea.

HOMEOPATHY

In homeopathy, substances are extensively diluted so that virtually no active substance is still present. The idea is that these substances are supposed to stimulate the body's own curative powers. There has been great controversy over the effectiveness of homeopathy. In reviewing various studies, some showed positive effects, while others revealed that homeopathy was no more effective for headaches than placebos. These treatments are very individualized, and one homeopathic remedy cannot be applied to all people. The drops are supposed to be taken every hour or two, and only for a limited period of time during the pain. Typical homeopathic remedies for headache include iris, belladonna, aconite, bryonia, gelsemium, and natrum muriaticum. Other remedies include sepia, sanguinaria, and *nux vomica*. These remedies are very safe. However, at this time the benefits of homeopathy for headaches remain unclear and unconvincing.

TRIGGER-POINT INJECTIONS

"Trigger points" are tender areas or areas of muscle tension just under the skin. When headaches are caused by muscle knots in the neck or head and are not easily relieved, trigger-point injections of Marcaine or lidocaine into the painful areas can be very effective, perhaps offering relief for weeks or even months. In some instances, doctors add cortisone, particularly for cluster headache or severe, long-lasting migraines. Certain pain centers give deeper injections, under fluoroscopy, in the hospital. This therapy might be beneficial, though it's not certain. Some people, however, will find the injections of no benefit. Recently, Botox (botulinum) injections have been used for prevention of headache; this remains in the experimental phase, but is promising.

Many patients with chronic daily headaches have fibromyalgia, and this can lead to all-too-familiar chronic neck pain and stiffness, with some tenderness. Injections of an anesthetic into these tender areas might help for a while.

However, injections are not a miracle cure, but then nothing is. Like other therapies to help pain, such as medications or physical therapy, injections can help ease the suffering for a period of time.

NERVE BLOCKS

Occipital nerve blocks, given in the back of the head, sound terrible but are actually safe and easy to do. These nerve blocks of anesthetic are sometimes used to relieve pain in the back of the head (occipital neuralgias). Many neurologists will do superficial blocks just under the skin, but some pain centers do "deep" blocks at the "root" of the occipital nerve. Each person has two occipital nerves, one on each side, and these contribute to headache pain. In fact, people with migraine have a 20 percent chance of having "occipital" neuralgia, or sharp pains around those nerves. Besides the usual medications for this problem (antidepressants, antiseizure medications), an injection near the occipital nerve can be helpful.

HYPNOSIS AND SELF-HYPNOSIS

Unfortunately, hypnosis has not been very helpful in treating headache. Biofeedback, a form of self-hypnosis, however, has been found to be quite beneficial. (See Chapter 2 for more details on biofeedback and other forms of self-hypnosis, such as imagery and relaxation techniques.)

ACUPUNCTURE

Acupuncture has been used to treat headaches for more than four thousand years. While not entirely conforming to modern scientific principles, acupuncture is helpful in some circumstances and is being used increasingly in the West. It is based on the principle of reestablishing a balance between the body's yin and yang. Easterners believe that these two opposing forces, representing feminine and masculine qualities, are at work in the human body and the cosmos.

Although we don't know exactly how or why acupuncture works, acupuncturists have identified about five hundred points that are related to nerve receptors. When stimulated, pain is somehow muted. Hair-thin stainless steel needles provide stimuli to the nervous system and work most effectively when applied to an area where nerve and muscle meet. Some American scientists suggest that acupuncture temporarily stimulates nerve cells to produce the body's natural painkillers, the enkephalins and endorphins. At least one study, using rats, conducted at the University of Texas Health Sciences Center, supports this theory.

The acupuncturist may insert the needles into selected points on the body's meridians — energy points considered essential to health. He or she may twirl the needles, stimulate them with mild electricity, or heat them to enhance the effectiveness of treatment. Electric stimulation seems to be the most effective mode.

Studies evaluating the efficacy of acupuncture for headaches are difficult to do, considering the high placebo response. The several studies that have been conducted produced conflicting findings for headaches, and the results of long-term studies have yet to come.

Although traditional Western physicians do not wholeheartedly endorse acupuncture, many doctors believe there is little harm in trying the services of a reputable (and in some states, licensed) acupuncturist. The procedure is generally very safe; occasionally side effects may occur, such as bleeding, faintness, or infection. The American Academy of Medical Acupuncture reports that some two thousand American physicians use acupuncture in their practices.

For more information and referrals, ask your doctor or medical center. (See Appendix A for specific addresses and phone numbers.) While acupuncture may produce short-term results, the effect tends to quickly wear off, and most people stop seeing the acupuncturist within weeks or months.

ACUPRESSURE

Acupressure involves applying circular finger pressure to some of the points that acupuncturists have identified. One acupressure point for headaches is the center of the web between your thumb and index finger. Apply pressure with the index finger from your other hand and, without lifting the finger, press in a circular motion. Other pressure points are the sides of the spine at the base of the neck.

For direct acupressure to the head, try rubbing your index fingers on the bony parts of your temples as close to the painful areas as possible, in small circles, pressing against the bone. Maintain the pressure for two minutes.

Other pressure points include the top of the ear; either side of the back of the neck at the base of the skull, where you can feel bony protrusions; and above your ears, where you can feel movement when you bite down. The effect is short-lived, and usually the pain returns when the acupuncture point is no longer stimulated.

TENS: TRANSCUTANEOUS ELECTRICAL
NERVE STIMULATION

A TENS unit is a battery-operated device that produces a small electrical current. Its pads are usually applied to the neck and lower skull to create a tingly, or vibrating, sensation. It may relieve some pain by blocking pain transmission signals or by stimulating the production of the body's own painkillers, endorphins. While TENS has some limited usefulness for chronic pain, such as low back pain, its ability to cure headaches has been very disappointing. The relief, if any, is very temporary. Some thought has been given to developing a TENS unit that is applied to the head and affects serotonin. Such a device was tested in the 1980s, and with more research it could be helpful in alleviating chronic headaches in the future.

CHIROPRACTIC MEASURES AND PHYSICAL THERAPY

Although not useful for many people, chiropractic treatment can be very helpful for some. It may include manipulation of the spine, ultrasound, diathermy (heat on the skin), deep heat, electrical stimulation, and massage. These therapies will help some headache patients, but overall, chiropractic measures appear to benefit the neck and back to a greater degree.

Physical therapists treat head and neck pain with the same techniques (with the exception of spine manipulation). As with chiropractic measures, physical therapy usually benefits the associated neck pain more than the head pain. It is particularly useful, however, after whiplash injuries, to improve posture, to relieve neck strain, and may help headaches caused by workstation strain.

MASSAGE AND STRETCHES

Massage to the neck and lower skull area benefits many headache sufferers by easing painful knots, but the benefits are usually short-lived. Full-body or face massages may help by relaxing you, whereas massaging the forehead, temple, back of the neck, and shoulders may be particularly useful for tension headaches. Craniosacral massage is particularly effective.

You can also relax these areas with some stretching exercises that involve the neck (rolling your head, gently pressing it forward with your hands at the base of your skull, rolling and shrugging your shoulders).

SEX

Believe it or not, sexual intercourse was found to help relieve migraines in about half the women studied in a research project at the Southern Illinois University School of Medicine. Men were not evaluated in the study, but for some the release of tension from intercourse just may help. However, sex or other exertion may also trigger headaches (see Chapter 13).

ICE OR HEAT

Applying cold (ice) to the head or heat to the neck have been mainstays of headache and neck-pain therapy for many years. Simply apply the cold to the area of head pain. Migraine Ice™ conveniently provides instant cold for headache or neck pain.

IMPROVING POSTURE

Positions that strain the neck, such as sitting at a computer for long periods, may contribute to headache pain. Adjust the seat and table so your neck is not bent or extended. Take breaks every fifteen minutes or so; do two minutes of stretching every two or three hours. Regular stretching of the neck and lower back can decrease headaches. Physical therapists can be very helpful for improving posture and teaching stretching.

MAGNETS (MAGNET THERAPY)

Magnets have been used for pain for decades, even centuries. They are a primary therapy for pain relief in Japan and are gaining popularity in the United States. Good studies on their use are beginning to trickle in, and they indicate that magnets are more beneficial for pain than a placebo. One study, published in the *American Journal of Psychiatry,* indicated a possible role for magnets in treating depression. We will not know definitively for years if magnets truly work better than placebos, though early results are encouraging. The lack of side effects and relative low cost, though, are very appealing. However, they should not be used if you or your partner has a cardiac pacemaker or other internal device. They should also not be used if pregnancy is a possibility.

The magnets are usually wrapped and placed about the head or neck for minutes to hours. Some people sleep on a magnet pillow or a bed with a mattress pad full of magnets. Several magnet companies make these products in convenient forms. There is no limit as to how long magnets can be left on. Magnets are primarily meant to treat pain that is already in progress (although they may prevent headache in some people).

The question as to why they may work has not yet been answered. One theory holds that they inhibit the firing of pain fibers in the skin, but they may influence neurotransmitters at deeper levels of the nervous system as well. These magnets are simple: north only, not bipolar, and low intensity (they will attract a paper clip somewhat, but do little more than that).

THE HEADACHE FRONTIER
• • • • • • • • • • • • • • • •

Most medications now used for headaches were developed for other purposes and then accidentally discovered to help headaches too. Chances are, some headache drugs of the future will be medications already on the market for other purposes.

Botulinum toxin (of which there are two types), for example, is a treatment for very severe muscle spasm. Injections may prove useful for chronic daily headaches when the muscles in the back of the head and neck are very tight. Injections in the muscles around the back of the head paralyze the muscles for three months, thereby providing some relief. It's still unclear if this treatment will hold up as a good therapy. For migraine or cluster headache prevention, ten to thirteen injections (mostly in the forehead area) have been used. Some people have had relief for up to four months. In the low doses used for headache, Botox is safe. For the acute treatment of migraine, intravenous Depacon (valproate) may assume a major role in the near future. Also, compounds in the brain, such as nitrous oxide, are being discovered to play a role in generating headaches. New therapies, based on these types of discoveries, are emerging. One new therapy, for example, may be as simple as using vitamin B_{12}, which decreases nitrous oxide.

In development, however, are new drugs that focus primarily on neurotransmitters in the brain. Serotonin has been widely investigated. Other therapies involving dopamine, vasoactive peptides, and nitrous oxide may prove helpful in the future.

The immune system may also be a fertile ground for new drug strategies. Scientists have uncovered evidence that a significant number of headache patients have lower numbers of immune cells called suppressors, implying an overactive immune system. Unrelated to allergies that are linked to the immune system, these cells counter the actions of helper cells in the immune response. Although certain drugs, such as the corticosteroids prednisone, Decadron, and Depo-Medrol, help migraine and cluster headaches for a brief time via the immune system, they have a wide array of side effects and their benefits tend to wane if used for long periods. The challenge is to develop safe but effective medications that alter the immune system in a way that helps headache patients and are deemed safe for long-term use. Singulair, a mild asthma medication, may be helpful as a migraine preventive.

As researchers get closer to discovering the gene that is responsible for inherited headaches, it may someday even be possible to alter genes to decrease migraine and tension headaches. Of course, scientists and patients must address many ethical and moral questions before undertaking gene therapy.

In the next thirty years, we will probably see more and more studies assessing the benefits of alternative treatments, such as herbs, sorting out which treatments are effective and worthwhile.

262 · HEADACHE HELP

PUTTING IT ALL TOGETHER
• • • • • • • • • • • • • • • • •

This book is chock full of advice and information that your doctor may consider for your headaches. We cannot stress strongly enough, however, that your own management techniques can go a very long way toward reducing the frequency and severity of headaches. To recap, we want to leave you with a roundup of suggestions:

- Recognize your headache problem as a legitimate physical illness. View and communicate your headache problem as if it were just like asthma, diabetes, or hypertension: an inherited physical, medical condition. Remember that a primary reason for your headaches is that you have too little serotonin in the brain. Acknowledge that because of a lack of serotonin, you may also have anxiety and depression.
- Help your doctor to achieve a balance between medication and headache pain. Your realistic goal is to improve the headaches 50 percent to 90 percent, while minimizing medications.
- Keep careful track of what medications (at what doses) did not work, what other conditions you have, and what other medications you take. In choosing preventives, your doctor will need to know if you suffer from any of these: anxiety, depression, insomnia, gastritis, heartburn, irritable bowel syndrome, constipation, hypertension, asthma, and sensitivities or allergies to other drugs. These often determine which way to proceed with medication. Include in this record any sensitivities or allergies to medications that you have ever had.
- Keep your own drug-medication chart. After a few years, you may have tried a dozen or two dozen different medications. Showing your doctor the chart at the beginning of treatment is immensely useful.
- You might become frustrated by the lack of effectiveness or by the side effects of daily preventives. Remember: 50 percent (at most) of patients achieve long-term relief with preventives.

Knowing this should allow you to realize that if they don't help, it's not your fault.

- You need to stick with preventive medications for at least four weeks (or longer); if you abandon them too soon, you may not see the beneficial effects.
- Consider psychotherapy. Although it won't necessarily improve your headaches, you can learn to cope better with headaches and the stresses that they produce. Unfortunately, because of stigma, time, and money, only a small minority of patients actually go to a therapist.
- If you have chronic daily headaches, understand that the "cure" may not be total. You may still have headaches every day, but they may be less severe. Ask yourself if you have gone from severe to moderate (from a "10" down to a "7") or from a moderate to a mild (from a "7" to a "4"). If you show improvement, all of the medication probably should not be changed.
- Be sure to tell your doctor how much OTC pain relief you use, including herbal preparations.
- Do not confuse addiction with dependency (see Chapter 5); when treating chronic daily headache, dependency has to be accepted.
- When nothing works: Don't give up! The end-of-the-line strategies include: MAOs, daily long-acting opioids (methadone, Kadian, Oxycontin), stimulants (dextroamphetamine, methylphenidate, phentermine), intravenous DHE, daily triptans in limited amounts, daily DHE (nasal spray), or combinations of approaches.
- Remember, good headache therapy, just like other challenges, requires patience, persistence, and perseverence.
- Learn how to cope with stress effectively, whether through cognitive strategies that can be learned from self-help books or in using relaxation and breathing techniques, exercise, yoga, massage, footbaths, or whatever works for you. Don't overload yourself with too many obligations. Learn to say no.
- Exercise regularly. Aerobic exercise — as little as twenty minutes of brisk walking three or four times a week — and daily neck and back stretches can help ward off headaches.

- Pay attention to your diet. Keep track of and limit foods that trigger your headaches. Eat regularly and healthfully (plenty of whole grains, pasta, fruits and vegetables; limit sugar, salt, and fat), do not skip meals, and drink a lot of water.
- Maintain a regular sleeping schedule. Try to wake up at the same time every day; sleeping late may trigger a headache.
- Avoid or limit alcohol, especially types that you know can trigger headaches.
- Control environmental factors that may trigger your headaches: avoid smoky rooms, fumes, and perfumes, for instance.
- See a doctor if you get headaches that interfere with your life.

APPENDICES

· · · · · · ·

INDEX

· · ·

·

APPENDIX A:
HEADACHE-RELATED
ORGANIZATIONS
AND PUBLICATIONS

· · · · · · · · · · · · · · · · ·

The following associations and foundations offer free or inexpensive materials on headaches.

FOR HEADACHE INFORMATION AND REFERRALS

> Visit Dr. Robbins's Web site at
> www.headachedrugs.com.

National Headache Foundation (NHF)
428 W. St. James Pl., 2nd Fl.
Chicago, IL 60614-2710
Tel: (800) 843-2256; Fax: (773) 525-7357
Web site: http://www.headaches.org
For $20 a year, you will receive a quarterly newsletter and access to the headache libraries.

American Council for Headache Education (ACHE)
19 Mantua Rd.
Mt. Royal, NJ 08061
Tel: (800) 255-ACHE
Web site: http://www.achenet.org
General information, help in starting a local headache support group, or referrals to members of the American Headache Society.

For $20 a year, you can subscribe to a quarterly newsletter on the latest developments in the headache field. On-line support: alt.support.headaches.migraine (newsgroup). Cluster headache: www.clusterheadaches.com.

TO START A HEADACHE SUPPORT GROUP

Sharing experiences and tips with others who face similar challenges can help you cope and feel more in control over your life and confident about your decisions.

ACHE and NHF (above) can both help. So can the following organization, which locates local self-help groups.

National Self-Help Clearinghouse
25 West 43rd St.
New York, NY 10036

Another organization that can help you find specific medical programs in your area:

American Self-Help Clearinghouse
St. Claire's Hospital
25 Pocono Rd.
Denville, NJ 07834
Tel: (973) 625-9665; Fax: (973) 625-8848
Web site: http://www.cmnc.com/selfhelp
E-mail: ashc@cybernex.net

HELP BY PHONE

To access medically oriented tape-recorded messages on medical topics, including relaxation and stress management, call: Health Messages, (888) 493-8300.

BIOFEEDBACK, RELAXATION, AND TAPES

Health Journeys, available on Time Warner AudioBooks: *For People with Headaches* (two-tape set).
Tapes by:

Belleruth Naparstek, Image Paths, Inc.
891 Moe Dr., Suite C
Akron, OH 44310
Tel: (800) 800-9661

The Source Cassette Learning System
Emmit Miller, M.D.
945 Evelyn St.
Menlo Park, CA 94025
Tel: (415) 328-7171

Association for Applied Psychophysiology and Biofeedback
10200 W. 44th Ave., Suite 304
Wheat Ridge, CO 80033-2840
Tel: (800) 477-8892; Fax: (303) 422-8894
Web site: http://aapb.org
E-mail: aapb@resourcenter.com

Quantum Quests
Box 986
Oakview, CA 93022
Tel: (800) 772-0090

Academy for Guided Imagery
P.O. Box 2070
Mill Valley, CA 94942
(800) 726-2070

International Imagery Association
P.O. Box 1046
Bronx, NY 10471

COUNSELING AND PSYCHOTHERAPY

American Psychiatric Association
1400 K St., NW
Washington, D.C. 20005
Tel: (202) 682-6000; Fax: (202) 682-6850
Web site: http://www.psych.org
E-mail: apa@psych.org

American Psychological Association
750 First St. NE
Washington, D.C. 20002-4242
Tel: (202) 336-5500; TDD (202) 336-6123;
Fax: (202) 336-5708
Web site: http://www.apa.org
E-mail: publiccom@apa.org

National Association of Social Workers
750 First St. NE, Suite 700
Washington, D.C. 20002
Tel: (202) 408-8600

Association for Advancement of Behavior Therapy (AABT)
305 Seventh Ave., Suite 1601
New York, NY 10001
Tel: (212) 647-1890; Fax: (212) 647-1865
Web site: http://www.aabt.org/aabt
E-mail: referral@aabt.org

Anxiety Disorders Association of America
11900 Parklawn Dr., Suite 100
Rockville, MD 20852-2624
Tel: (301) 231-9350; Fax: (301) 231-7392
Web site: http://www.adaa.org
E-mail: anxdis@aol.com

Anxiety Disorder Education Program/National Institute of
    Mental Health
5600 Fishers Lane, Rm. 7C-02
Rockville, MD 20857
Tel: (800) 647-2642
Web site: http://www.nimh.nih.gov/anxiety/index.htm
E-mail: nimhinfo@nih.gov

National Anxiety Foundation
3135 Custer Dr.
Lexington, KY 40517
Web site: http://www.lexington-on-line.com/naf.html

Depression and Related Affective Disorders Association
    (DRADA)
Meyer 3-181, 600 N. Wolfe St.
Baltimore, MD 21287-7381
Tel: (410) 955-4647; Fax: (410) 614-3241
Web site: http://www.med.jhu.edu/drada
E-mail: drada@welchlink.welch.jhu.edu

National Depressive and Manic-Depressive Association
730 N. Franklin, #501
Chicago, IL 60610
Tel: (800) 826-3632; Fax: (312) 642-7243
Web site: http://www.ndmda.org
E-mail: myrtis@aol.com

National Foundation for Depressive Illness
P.O. Box 2257
New York, NY 10116
Tel: (800) 239-1298
Web site: http://www.depression.org

National Mental Health Association
1021 Prince St.
Alexandria, VA 22314
Tel: (800) 969-6642; TTY: (800) 433-5959;
Fax: (703) 684-5968
Web site: http://nmha.org
E-mail: nmhainfo@aol.com

Depression Awareness Recognition and Treatment Education
    Program (DART)
National Institute of Mental Health
5600 Fishers Lane
Rockville, MD 20857
Tel: (800) 421-4211 (free brochures)
Web site: http://www.nimh.nih.gov/dart/darthome.htm

Obsessive-Compulsive Foundation
9 Depot St., P.O. Box 70
Milford, CT 06460
Tel: (203) 878-5669: Fax: (203) 874-2826
Web site: http://www.ocfoundation.org
E-mail: info@ocfoundation.org

HERBS

American Herb Association
Box 353
Rescue, CA 95672

Herb Research Foundation
1007 Pearl Street, Suite 200
Boulder, CO 80302
Tel: (800) 748-2617

Herbal Green Pages 1995–1996
Herb Growing & Marketing Network
P.O. Box 245
Silver Springs, PA 17575
Tel: (717) 393-3295

The Herb Companion Wishbook and Resource Guide, by
        Bobbie McRae
Interweave Press
Box 49770
Austin, TX 78765-9770

Herb Society of America
9019 Kirtland Chardon Rd.
Kirtland, OH 44094
Tel: (440) 256-0514

American Botanical Council
P.O. Box 201660
Austin, TX 78720
Tel: (800) 373-7105

AROMATHERAPY

Pacific Institute of Aromatherapy
P.O. Box 6723
San Rafael, CA 94903
Tel: (415) 479-9121

Essence Aromatherapy
P.O. Box 2119
Durango, CO 81302
Tel: (800) 283-0244

Aromatherapy Quarterly
P.O. Box 421
Inverness, CA 94937
Tel: (415) 669-7378

Floralis
P.O. Box 40233
Washington, D.C. 20016
Tel: (781) 861-6142

FIBROMYALGIA AND CHRONIC PAIN

American Chronic Pain Association
P.O. Box 850
Rocklin, CA 95677
Tel: (916) 632-0922

International Association for the Study of Pain
Seattle, WA
Tel: (206) 547-6409

Fibromyalgia Network
P.O. Box 31750
Tucson, AZ 85751
Tel: (800) 853-2929; Fax: (520) 290-5550
Web site: http://www.fmnetnews.com

ALTERNATIVE AND NATUROPATHIC MEDICINE

Office of Alternative Medicine
National Institutes of Health
Information Center
6120 Executive Blvd., Suite 450
Rockville, MD 20892-9904
Tel: (301) 402-2466

Center for Alternative Medicine Clearinghouse
P.O. Box 8218
Silver Spring, MD 20907-8218
Tel: (888) 644-6226

American Holistic Medical Association
433 Front St.
Catasauqua, PA 18032
Tel: (610) 433-2448

American Association of Naturopathic Physicians
P.O. Box 2579
Kirkland, WA 98083-2579

National College of Naturopathic Medicine
11231 Southeast Market Street
Portland, OR 97216
Tel: (503) 255-4860

Mind-Body Medical Institute
110 Francis St., Suite 1A
Boston, MA 02215
Tel: (617) 632-9530

Center for Mind-Body Medicine
5225 Connecticut Ave., N.W., Suite 414
Washington, D.C. 20015
Tel: (202) 966-7338

ACUPUNCTURE AND ACUPRESSURE

Acupressure Institute
1533 Shattuck Ave.
Berkeley, CA 94709
Tel: (800) 442-2232, (510) 845-1059

American Oriental Bodywork Association
6801 Jericho Turnpike
Syosset, NY 11791
Tel: (516) 364-5533

American Academy of Medical Acupuncture
Tel: (800) 521-2262

American Association of Acupuncture and Oriental Medicine
433 Front St.
Catasauqua, PA 18032
Tel: (610) 266-1433; Fax: (610) 264-2768

CHINESE MEDICINE

American Foundation of Traditional Chinese Medicine
505 Beach St.
San Francisco, CA 94133
Tel: (415) 776-0502

Blue Poppy Press
1775 Linden Ave.
Boulder, CO 80304
Tel: (800) 487-9296
Publishes a variety of books on traditional Chinese medicine

Insight Publishing
Box 18476
Anaheim Hills, CA 92817
Tel: (800) 787-2600
Catalog of books on traditional Chinese medicine

OSTEOPATHY, CRANIOSACRAL THERAPY, AND MASSAGE

American Osteopathic Association
142 East Ontario St.
Chicago, IL 60611
Tel: (800) 621-1773
In Illinois: (312) 280-5800

American Academy of Osteopathy
3500 DePauw Boulevard, Suite 1080
Indianapolis, IN 46268
Tel: (317) 879-1881

The Cranial Academy
8202 Clear Vista Parkway, #9D
Indianapolis, IN 46256
Tel: (317) 594-0411

American Massage Therapy Association
820 Davis St., Suite 100
Evanston, IL 60201
Tel: (847) 864-0123

HYPNOSIS

American Institute of Hypnotherapy
16842 VonKarman Ave., Suite 475
Irvine, CA 92714
Tel: (949) 261-6400

American Society for Clinical Hypnosis
33 W. Grand Ave., Suite 402
Chicago, IL 60610
Tel: (312) 645-9810

YOGA

Himalayan Institute of Yoga, Science, and Philosophy
R.R. 1, Box 400
Honesdale, PA 18431
Tel: (570) 253-5551, (800) 822-4547

International Association of Yoga Therapists
P.O. Box 1386
Lower Lake, CA 95457
Tel: (707) 928-9898

SLEEP DISORDERS

Narcolepsy Network
277 Fairfield Rd., Suite 310B
Fairfield, NJ 07004
Tel: (973) 276-0115; Fax (973) 227-8224
Web site: http://www.websciences.org/narnet
E-mail: NARNET@aol.com

American Sleep Disorders Association
6301 Bandel Rd., #101
Rochester, MN 55901
Tel: (507) 287-6006; Fax: (507) 287-6008
Web site: http://www.asda.org
E-mail: asda@asda.org

National Sleep Foundation
729 15th St., NW, 4th Fl.
Washington, D.C. 20005
Tel: (888) 637-7533; Fax: (202) 347-3472
Web site: http://www.sleepfoundation.org
E-mail: natsleep@erols.com

BRAIN AND HEAD INJURIES

Brain Injury Association
105 N. Alfred St.
Alexandria, VA 22314
Tel: (800) 444-6443; Fax: (703) 236-6001
Web site: http://www.biausa.org
E-mail: FamilyHelpline@biausa.org

Head Injury Hotline
212 Pioneer Bldg.
Seattle, WA 98104-2221
Tel: (206) 621-8558; Fax: (206) 624-4961
Web site: http://www.headinjury.com
E-mail: brain@headinjury.com

ATTENTION DEFICIT DISORDER (ADD)

Children and Adults with Attention Deficit Disorders (CHADD)
499 NW 70th Ave., Suite 101
Plantation, FL 33317
Tel: (800) 233-4050; Fax: (954) 587-4599
Web site: http://www.chadd.org
E-mail: national@chadd.org

CHIROPRACTIC

American Chiropractic Association
1701 Clarendon Boulevard
Arlington, VA 22209
Tel: (703) 276-8800

International Chiropractors Association
1110 North Glebe Rd., Suite 1000
Arlington, VA 22201
Tel: (703) 528-5000

BRAIN TUMORS AND NEUROLOGICAL DISORDERS

Institute for Brain and Immune Disorders
914 South 8th St.
Minneapolis, MN 55404
Tel: (612) 337-8953; Fax: (612) 347-3915
Web site: http://www.winternet.com/~briminst
E-mail: igarao01@tc.umn.edu

National Institute of Neurological Disorders and Stroke
Office of Scientific and Health Reports
P.O. Box 5801
Bethesda, MD 20824
Tel: (800) 352-9424
Web site: http://www.ninds.nih.gov

National Brain Tumor Foundation
785 Market St., Suite 1600
San Francisco, CA 94103
Tel: (800) 934-2873; Fax: (415) 284-0209
Web site: http://www.braintumor.org
E-mail: nbtf@braintumor.org

APPENDIX B:
OVER-THE-COUNTER
HEADACHE MEDICATIONS

. . . .

The following table lists the most common over-the-counter headache medications and their composition. You may compare medications, for example, by their caffeine content and whether they contain acetaminophen or aspirin. By knowing how much of a compound these medications contain, you can compare their relative strength and their likelihood of giving you discomfort if you are sensitive, for example, to aspirin.

Note: Pseudoephedrine is a vasoconstrictor (blood vessel constrictor) of the upper respiratory tract; as a result, it helps shrink swollen tissues in the sinuses and nose.

OVER-THE-COUNTER HEADACHE MEDICATIONS

Brand-name Medication	Aspirin	Acetaminophen	Ibuprofen	Caffeine	Pseudoephedrine	Other
Aspirin Free Anacin Caplets		500 mg				
Aspirin Free Anacin Tablets		500 mg				
Aspirin Free Anacin P.M. Caplets		500 mg				diphenhydramine hydrochloride 25 mg
Aspirin Free Excedrin Analgesic Caplets		500 mg		65 mg		
Excedrin Extra-Strength Analgesic Tablets and Caplets	250 mg	250 mg		65 mg		
Excedrin P.M. Analgesic/Sleeping Aid		500 mg				diphenhydramine citrate 38 mg
Maximum Strength Multi-Symptom Menstrual Formula Midol		500 mg		60 mg		pyrilamine maleate 15 mg
PMS Multi-Symptom Formula Midol		500 mg				parabrom 25 mg pyrilamine maleate 15 mg
Regular Strength Multi-Symptom Midol Formula		325 mg				pyrilamine maleate 15 mg
Multi-Symptom Pamprin Tablets and Caplets		500 mg				parabrom 25 mg pyrilamine maleate 15 mg
Maximum Pain Relief Pamprin Caplets		250 mg				magnesium salicylate 250 mg, parabrom 25 mg
Maximum Strength Panadol Tablets and Caplets		500 mg				
Percogesic Analgesic Tablets		325 mg				phenyltoloxamine citrate 30 mg
Sominex Pain Relief Formula		500 mg				diphenhydramine hydrochloride 25 mg

Brand-name Medication	Aspirin	Aceta-minophen	Ibuprofen	Caffeine	Pseudo-ephedrine	Other
St. Joseph Aspirin-Free Fever Reducer for Children Chewable Tablets		80 mg				
Tylenol Children's Chewable Tablets, Elixir, and Suspension Liquid		Tablets 80 mg; Elixir 160 mg (5 ml); Liquid 160 mg (5 ml)				
Tylenol Extra Strength, Adult Liquid Pain Reliever		15 ml–500 mg				
Tylenol Extra Strength, Gelcaps, Caplets, and Tablets		500 mg				
Tylenol Junior Strength, Coated Caplets, Grape and Fruit Chewable Tablets		160 mg				
Tylenol Regular Strength, Caplets and Tablets		325 mg				
Tylenol PM Extra Strength Pain Reliever/ Sleep Aid Gelcaps, Caplets, and Tablets		500 mg				diphenhydramine hydrochloride 25 mg
Unisom with Pain Relief Nighttime Sleep Aid/Analgesic		650 mg				diphenhydramine hydrochloride 50 mg
Vanquish Analgesic Caplets	227 mg	194 mg		33 mg		dried aluminum hydroxide gel 25 mg, magnesium hydroxide 50 mg
Tylenol Headache Plus Pain Reliever with Antacid Caplets		500 mg				calcium carbonate 250 mg
Bayer Children's Chewable Aspirin	81 mg					

Brand-name Medication	Aspirin	Aceta-minophen	Ibuprofen	Caffeine	Pseudo-ephedrine	Other
Genuine Bayer Aspirin Tablets and Caplets	325 mg					hydroxypropyl methylcellulose coating for easier swallowing
Maximum Bayer Aspirin Tablets and Caplets	500 mg					hydroxypropyl methylcellulose coating for easier swallowing
Extended Release Bayer 8-Hour Aspirin	650 mg					
Adult Low Strength Enteric Aspirin Tablets	81 mg					
Regular Strength Bayer Enteric Aspirin Caplets	325 mg					
Empirin Aspirin	325 mg					
Norwich Aspirin	325 mg					
Norwich Aspirin Maximum Strength	500 mg					
Arthritis Pain Formula	500 mg					
Aspergum	227 mg					
Goody's Extra Strength	260 mg	130 mg		16.25 mg		
Goody's Extra Strength Headache	520 mg	260 mg		32.5 mg		
Norwich Enteric Safety Coated Aspirin	325 mg					
Norwich Enteric Safety Coated Aspirin Maximun Strength	500 mg					
St. Joseph Adult Chewable Aspirin	81 mg					
Anacin Caplets	400 mg			32 mg		
Anacin Tablets	400 mg			32 mg		
Maximum Strength Anacin Tablets	500 mg			32 mg		
Arthritis Strength BC Powder	742 mg			36 mg		salicylamide 222 mg
Ascriptin A/D Caplets	325 mg					buffered with Maalox (alumina-magnesia) and calcium carbonate

Brand-name Medication	Aspirin	Aceta-minophen	Ibuprofen	Caffeine	Pseudo-ephedrine	Other
Extra Strength Ascriptin Caplets	500 mg					buffered with Maalox (alumina-magnesia) and calcium carbonate
Regular Strength Ascriptin Caplets	325 mg					buffered with Maalox (alumina-magnesia) and calcium carbonate
BC Powder	650 mg			32 mg		salicylamide 195 mg
BC Cold Powder Multi-Symptom Formula (Cold-Sinus-Allergy)	650 mg					phenylpropano-lamine hydrochloride 25 mg, chlorphenira-mine maleate 4 mg
BC Cold Powder Non-Drowsy Formula (Cold-Sinus)	650 mg					phenylpropano-lamine hydrochlo-ride 25 mg
Bayer Plus Aspirin Tablets	325 mg					buffered with calcium carbonate, magne-sium carbonate, magnesium oxide
Extra Strength Bayer Plus Aspirin Caplets	500 mg					buffered with calcium carbonate, magne-sium carbonate, magnesium oxide
Arthritis Strength Bufferin Analgesic Caplets	500 mg					buffered with calcium carbonate, magne-sium carbonate, magnesium oxide
Extra Strength Bufferin Analgesic Tablets	500 mg					buffered with calcium carbonate, magne-sium carbonate, magnesium oxide
Bufferin Analgesic Tablets and Caplets	325 mg					buffered with calcium carbonate, magne-sium carbonate, magnesium oxide
Ecotrin Enteric Coated Aspirin Maximum Strength Tablets and Caplets	500 mg					acetylsalicylic acid
Ecotrin Enteric Coated Aspirin Regular Strength Tablets and Caplets	325 mg					acetylsalicylic acid

Brand-name Medication	Aspirin	Aceta-minophen	Ibuprofen	Caffeine	Pseudo-ephedrine	Other
Excedrin Extra-Strength Analgesic Tablets and Caplets	250 mg	250 mg		65 mg		
BC Tablet	325 mg					
BC Arthritis Strength	742 mg			36 mg		
Cope	421 mg			32 mg		
P-A-C Analgesic Tablets	400 mg			caffeine anhy-drous 32 mg		
Vanquish Analgesic Caplets	227 mg	194 mg		33 mg		dried aluminum hy-droxide gel 25 mg, magnesium hydroxide 50 mg
Aleve Tablets						naproxen 220 mg
Alka-Seltzer Efferve-scent Antacid and Pain Reliever	325 mg					heat-treated sodium bicarbon-ate 1916 mg, citric acid 1000 mg
Alka-Seltzer Extra Strength Efferves-scent Antacid and Pain Reliever	500 mg					heat-treated sodium bicarbon-ate 1985 mg, citric acid 1000 mg
Alka-Seltzer (Flavored) Effervescent Antacid and Pain Reliever	325 mg					heat-treated sodium bicarbon-ate 1710 mg, citric acid 1220 mg
Regular Strength Ascriptin Tablets	325 mg					buffered with Maalox (alumina-magnesia) and calcium carbonate
Advil Ibuprofen Caplets and Tablets			200 mg			
Bayer Select Ibu-profen Pain Relief Formula			200 mg			
Haltran Tablets			200 mg			
Ibuprohm Ibuprofen Caplets			200 mg			
Ibuprohm Ibuprofen Tablets			200 mg			
Doan's Extra Strength						magnesium salicylate 500 mg

Brand-name Medication	Aspirin	Aceta-minophen	Ibuprofen	Caffeine	Pseudo-ephedrine	Other
Doan's Regular Strength						magnesium salicylate 377 mg
Motrin, Children's			100 mg per 5 ml			
Motrin IB Caplets and Tablets			200 mg			
Nuprin Ibuprofen/ Analgesic Tablets and Caplets			200 mg			
Extra Strength Doan's P.M.						magnesium salicylate 500 mg, diphenhydra-mine hydrochloride 25 mg
Mobigesic Analgesic Tablets						magnesium salicylate 325 mg, phenyltolox-amine citrate 30 mg
Actifed Plus Caplets		500 mg			30 mg	triprolidine hydro-chloride 1.25 mg
Actifed Plus Tablets		500 mg			30 mg	triprolidine hydro-chloride 1.25 mg
Actifed Sinus Daytime/Nighttime Caplets		Daytime 325 mg, Night-time 500 mg			Daytime 30 mg, Night-time 30 mg	diphenhydramine hydrochloride 25 mg
Actifed Sinus Daytime/Nighttime Tablets		Daytime 325 mg, Night-time 500 mg			Daytime 30 mg, Night-time 30 mg	diphenhydramine hydrochloride 25 mg
Advil Cold and Sinus (formerly CoAdvil)			200 mg		30 mg	
Chlor-Trimeton Allergy-Sinus Headache Caplets		500 mg				chlorpheniramine maleate 2 mg, phenylpropanolamine hydrochloride, 12.5 mg
OrudisKT						ketoprofen 12.5 mg
Ketoprofen (generic)						ketoprofen 12.5 mg
Valprin		200 mg				

Brand-name Medication	Aspirin	Aceta-minophen	Ibuprofen	Caffeine	Pseudo-ephedrine	Other
Comtrex Multi-Symptom Cold Reliever Tablets, Caplets, Liqui-gels, and Liquid		Tablet 325 mg, Caplet 325 mg, Liqui-gel 325 mg, Liquid 650 mg			Tablet 30 mg, Caplet 30 mg, Liquid 60 mg	phenylpropanolamine hydrochloride (Liqui-gel only) 12.5 mg chlorpheniramine maleate (Tablet, Caplet, and Liqui-gel 2 mg, Liquid 4 mg) dextromethorphan (Tablet, Caplet, and Liqui-gel 10 mg, Liquid 20 mg)
Comtrex Multi-Symptom Non-Drowsy Caplets		325 mg			30 mg	dextromethorphan hydrobromide 10 mg
Dimetapp Sinus Caplets			200 mg		30 mg	
Dristan Sinus			200 mg		30 mg	
Sinus Excedrin Analgesic Decon-gestant Tablets and Caplets		500 mg			30 mg	
Sinarest No Drowsiness Tablets		500 mg			30 mg	
Sinarest Tablets		325 mg			30 mg	chlorpheniramine maleate 2 mg
Sinarest Extra Strength Tablets		500 mg			30 mg	chlorpheniramine maleate 2 mg
Sine-Aid Maxi-mum Strength Sinus Headache Gelcaps, Caplets, and Tablets		500 mg			30 mg	
Sine-Off Maximum Strength No Drowsiness Formula Caplets			500 mg		30 mg	
Sine-Off Sinus Medi-cine Tablets Aspirin Formula	325 mg					chlorpheniramine maleate 2 mg phenylpropanolamine hydrochloride 12.5 mg

Brand-name Medication	Aspirin	Aceta-minophen	Ibuprofen	Caffeine	Pseudo-ephedrine	Other
Sinutab Sinus Allergy Medication, Maximum Strength Caplets		500 mg			30 mg	chlorpheniramine maleate 2 mg
Sinutab Sinus Medication, Maximum Strength without Drowsiness Formula, Tablets and Caplets		500 mg			30 mg	
Sinutab Sinus Medication, Regular Strength without Drowsiness Formula		325 mg			30 mg	
Sudafed Plus Tablets					60 mg	chlorpheniramine maleate 4 mg
Sudafed Sinus Caplets		500 mg			30 mg	
Tylenol Allergy Sinus Medication Maximum Strength Gelcaps and Caplets		500 mg			30 mg	chlorpheniramine maleate 2 mg
Tylenol Cold Medication No Drowsiness Formula Gelcaps and Caplets		325 mg			30 mg	dextromethorphan hydrobromide 15 mg
Tylenol Cold Night Time Medication		650 mg/ 30 ml			60 mg/ 30 ml	diphenhydramine hydrochloride 50 mg/30 ml
Tylenol, Maximum Strength, Sinus Medication Gelcaps, Caplets, and Tablets		500 mg			30 mg	
Benadryl Allergy Sinus Headache Formula		500 mg			30 mg	diphenhydramine hydrochloride 12.5 mg
Allergy-Sinus Comtrex Multi-Symptom Allergy-Sinus Formula Tablets and Caplets		500 mg			30 mg	chlorpheniramine maleate 2 mg
Sinus Excedrin Analgesic, Decongestant Tablets and Caplets		500 mg			30 mg	

Brand-name Medication	Aspirin	Aceta-minophen	Ibuprofen	Caffeine	Pseudo-ephedrine	Other
BRAND-NAME ANTINAUSEA MEDICATION						
Dramamine Chewable Tablets						dimenhydrinate 50 mg
Dramamine Tablets						dimenhydrinate 50 mg
Emetrol						5 ml teaspoonful: dextrose 1.87 g, levulose 1.87 g, phosphor acid 21.5 mg
Marezine Tablets						cyclizine hydrochloride 50 mg
Pepto-Bismol Liquid						15 ml: bismuth subsalicylate 262 mg, salicylate 130 mg
Pepto-Bismol Tablets						bismuth subsalicylate 262 mg, salicylate 102 mg

APPENDIX C:
MEDICATIONS AND
WHAT'S IN THEM

. . . .

Brand Name	Composition
Actifed Allergy Daytime	Caplets: 30 mg pseudoephedrine
Actifed Allergy Nighttime	Caplets: 30 mg pseudoephedrine, 25 mg diphenhydramine
Actifed Cold and Allergy	Tablets: 60 mg pseudoephedrine, 2.5 mg triprolidine
Actifed Cold and Sinus	Caplets, Tablets: 500 mg acetaminophen, 30 mg pseudoephedrine, 1.25 mg triprolidine
Actifed Sinus Daytime	Caplets, Tablets: 500 mg acetaminophen, 30 mg pseudoephedrine
Adderall	Tablets: 10 mg, 20 mg dextroamphetamine with amphetamine
Adipex-P	Capsules, Tablets: 37.5 mg phentermine
Advil	Caplets, Gelcaps, Tablets: 200 mg ibuprofen Liquid: 100 mg/5ml ibuprofen
Advil, Children's	Chewable Tablets: 50 mg ibuprofen Suspension: 100 mg/5 ml ibuprofen Drops: 50 mg/1.25 ml ibuprofen
Aldactone	Tablets: 25 mg, 50 mg, 100 mg spironolactone

Brand Name	Composition
Alesse-21	
Alesse-28	Tablets: 0.10 mg levonorgestrel, 0.02 mg ethinyl estradiol
Aleve	Caplets, Tablets: 220 mg naproxen sodium
Alka Seltzer Effervescent, Original	Tablets: 1000 mg citric acid, 1916 mg sodium bicarbonate, 325 mg aspirin
Alka Seltzer Plus, Sinus	Tablets: 20 mg phenyl-propanolamine, 325 mg aspirin
Allerest Headache Strength Advanced Formula	Tablets: 30 mg pseudoephedrine, 2 mg chlorpheniramine, 325 mg aspirin
Altace	Capsules: 1.25 mg, 2.5 mg, 5 mg, 10 mg ramipril
Ambien	Tablets: 5 mg, 10 mg zolpidem tartrate
Amerge	Tablets: 1 mg, 2.5 mg naratriptan
amitriptyline (*see* Elavil)	
Anacin	Caplets, Gelcaps, Tablets: 400 mg aspirin, 32 mg caffeine
Anacin, Aspirin Free	Caplets, Gelcaps, Tablets: 500 mg acetaminophen
Anacin Maximum Strength	Caplets, Tablets: 500 mg aspirin, 32 mg caffeine
Anacin PM, Aspirin Free	Caplets, Gelcaps, Tablets: 500 mg acetaminophen, 25 mg diphenhydramine
Anaprox	Tablets: 275 mg naproxen sodium
Anaprox DS	Tablets: 550 mg naproxen sodium
Androderm Transdermal System	Patch: 2.5 mg/day, 5 mg/day testosterone
Ansaid	Tablets: 50 mg, 100 mg flurbiprofen
Antivert	Tablets: 12.5 mg meclizine
Antivert/25	Tablets: 25 mg meclizine
Antivert/50	Tablets: 50 mg meclizine

Brand Name	Composition
Arthritis Pain Formula	Tablets: 500 mg aspirin, 27 mg aluminum hydroxide, 100 mg magnesium hydroxide
Arthrotec	Tablets: 50 mg diclofenac, 200 mcg misoprostol, 75 mg diclofenac, 200 mcg misoprostol
Ativan	Tablets: 0.5 mg, 1 mg, 2 mg lorazepam
	Injection: 2 mg/ml, 4 mg/ml lorazepam
Aventyl	Capsules: 10 mg, 25 mg nortriptyline
Axid	Capsules: 150 mg, 300 mg nizatidine
Axocet	Capsules: 650 mg acetaminophen, 50 mg butalbital
Bancap HC	Tablets: 500 mg acetaminophen, 5 mg hydrocodone
Bayer Aspirin	Caplets, Tablets: 325 mg aspirin
Bayer Children's Aspirin	Chewable tablets: 81 mg aspirin
Bayer Enteric Aspirin	Enteric coated tablets: 81 mg aspirin Enteric coated caplets: 325 mg aspirin
Bayer Maximum Aspirin	Caplets, Tablets: 500 mg aspirin
Bayer Select Maximum Strength Headache	Caplets, Tablets: 500 mg aspirin, 65 mg caffeine
Bayer Timed Release Aspirin	Caplets, Tablets: 650 mg aspirin
BC Headache Powders	Powder: 650 mg aspirin, 32 mg caffeine, 195 mg salicylamide
Benadryl Allergy Kapseal	Capsules: 25 mg diphenhydramine
Benadryl Allergy Ultratabs	Tablets: 25 mg diphenhydramine
Benadryl Allergy Liquid	Suspension: 12.5 mg diphenhydramine

Brand Name	Composition
Bentyl	Capsules: 10 mg dicyclomine Tablets: 20 mg dicyclomine Syrup: 10 mg/5 ml dicyclomine Injection: 10 mg/ml dicyclomine
Blocadren	Tablets: 5 mg, 10 mg, 20 mg timolol maleate
bromocriptine (*see* Parlodel)	
Bromo Seltzer	Effervescent granules: 2781 mg sodium bicarbonate, 325 mg acetaminophen, 2224 mg citric acid
Bufferin	Tablets: 325 mg aspirin, 158 mg calcium carbonate, 63 mg magnesium oxide, 34 mg magnesium carbonate
Bumex	Tablets: 0.5 mg, 1 mg, 2 mg bumetanide Injection: 0.25 mg/ml bumetanide
Buspar	Tablets: 5 mg, 10 mg buspirone Dividose tablets: 15 mg buspirone
Cafergot (available as generic also: Belcomp, Ercaf, Ergocaf, Micomp)	Tablets: 1 mg ergotamine, 100 mg caffeine
Cafergot PB (adds pentobarbital and belladonna to above)	Suppositories: 2 mg ergotamine, 100 mg caffeine
Calan	Tablets: 40 mg, 80 mg, 120 mg verapamil
Calan SR	Caplets: 120 mg, 180 mg, 240 mg verapamil
Cardizem	Tablets: 30 mg, 60 mg, 90 mg, 120 mg diltiazem
Cardizem SR	SR Capsules: 60 mg, 90 mg, 120 mg diltiazem
Cardizem CD	Extended Release Capsules: 120 mg, 180 mg, 240 mg, 300 mg diltiazem
Catapres	Tablets: 0.1 mg, 0.2 mg, 0.3 mg clonidine

Brand Name	Composition
Catapres-TTS1 Transdermal Therapeutic System	Patch: 0.1 mg/day clonidine
Catapres-TTS2 Transdermal Therapeutic System	Patch: 0.2 mg/day clonidine
Catapres-TTS3 Transdermal Therapeutic System	Patch: 0.3 mg/day clonidine
Celebrex	Capsules: 100 mg, 200 mg celecoxib
Celexa	Tablets: 20 mg, 40 mg citalopram
Claritin	Tablets (Reditabs): 10 mg loratidine
Claritin-D 12 Hour	Tablets: 5 mg loratidine, 120 mg pseudoephedrine
Claritin-D 24 Hour	Tablets: 10 mg loratidine, 240 mg pseudoephedrine
Compazine	Tablets: 5 mg, 10 mg, 25 mg prochlorperazine maleate Spansules: 10 mg, 15 mg prochlorperazine maleate Suppositories: 2.5 mg, 5 mg, 25 mg prochlorperazine maleate Injection: 5 mg/ml prochlorperazine maleate
Comtrex Allergy Sinus	Tablets: 2 mg chlorpheniramine, 500 mg acetaminophen, 30 mg pseudoephedrine
Contac 12 Hour	Capsules: 75 mg phenyl-propanolamine, 8 mg chlorpheniramine
Contac Maximum Strength 12 Hour	Capsules: 75 mg phenylpropanolamine, 12 mg chlorpheniramine
Corgard	Tablets: 20 mg, 40 mg, 80 mg, 120 mg, 160 mg nadolol
Covera HS	Tablets: 180 mg, 240 mg verapamil
Cozaar	Tablets: 25 mg, 50 mg losartan potassium
Crinone	Cream: 4%, 8% progesterone
Cylert	Tablets: 18.75 mg, 37.5 mg, 75 mg pemoline Chewable Tablets: 37.5 mg pemoline

Brand Name	Composition
cyproheptadine (*see* Periactin)	
Cystospaz	Tablets: 0.15 mg hyoscyamine
Cystospaz-M	Capsules: 0.375 mg hyoscyamine sulfate
Cytomel	Tablets: 5 mcg, 25 mcg, 50 mcg liothyronine mesylate
Dallergy	Caplets: 8 mg chlorpheniramine, 20 mg phenylephrine, 1.25 mg methscopolamine
Dalmane	Capsules: 15 mg, 30 mg flurazepam
Darvocet N-100	Tablets: 100 mg propoxyphene napsylate, 325 mg acetaminophen
Darvon N	Tablets: 100 mg propoxyphene napsylate
Darvon	Pulvule: 65 mg propoxyphene
Darvon Compound-65	Pulvules: 65 mg propoxyphene, 389 mg aspirin, 32.4 mg caffeine
Daypro	Caplets: 600 mg oxaprozin
Decadron	Tablets: 0.25 mg, 0.5 mg, 0.75 mg, 1.5 mg, 4 mg, 6 mg dexamethasone
Deltasone	Tablets: 2.5 mg, 5 mg, 10 mg, 20 mg, 50 mg prednisone
Demerol	Tablets: 50 mg, 100 mg meperidine
Demulen 1/50	Tablets: 1 mg ethynodiol acetate, 50 mg ethinyl estradiol
Depacon injection	100 mg/ml valproate sodium
Depakote	Delayed Release Tablets: 125 mg, 250 mg, 500 mg divalproex sodium Sprinkle Capsules: 125 mg divalproex sodium
Depo-Medrol	Injection: 20 mg/ml, 40 mg/ml, 80 mg/ml methylprednisolone acetate
Desyrel	Tablets: 50 mg, 100 mg trazodone Dividose Tablets: 150 mg, 300 mg trazodone

Brand Name	Composition
Dexedrine	Tablets: 5 mg dextroamphetamine sulfate Spansules: 5 mg, 10 mg, 15 mg dextroamphetamine sulfate
DHE 45	Injection: 1 mg/ml dihydroergotamine mesylate
Diamox	Tablets: 125 mg, 250 mg acetazolamide Extended Release Capsules: 500 mg acetazolamide Injection: 500 mg/vial acetazolamide
diazepam (*see* Valium)	
Dilantin	Suspension: 30 mg/5 ml, 125 mg/5 ml phenytoin Injection: 50 mg/ml phenytoin Chewable Tablets: 50 mg phenytoin Extended Release Capsules: 100 mg phenytoin
Dilaudid	Syrup: 1 mg/5 ml hydromorphone Tablets: 1 mg, 2 mg, 3 mg, 4 mg hydromorphone Injection: 2 mg/ml, 3 mg/ml, 4 mg/ml, 10 mg/ml hydromorphone Suppositories: 3 mg hydromorphone
Disalcid	Capsules: 500 mg salsalate Tablets: 500 mg, 750 mg salsalate
Ditropan	Tablets: 5 mg oxybutynin chloride Syrup: 5 mg/5 ml oxybutynin chloride
Dolobid	Tablets: 250 mg, 500 mg diflunisal
Dolophine (*see* Methadone)	
Donnatal	Tablets: 16.2 mg phenobarbital, 0.137 hyoscyamine, 0.194 mg atropine, 0.0065 mg scopolamine Capsules: 16.2 mg phenobarbital, 0.137 mg hyoscyamine, 0.194 mg atropine, 0.0065 mg scopolamine
Doral	Tablet: 7.5 mg, 15 mg quazepam

Brand Name	Composition
droperidol	Injection: 2.5 mg/ml droperidol
Dristan Cold	Caplets, Tablets: 500 mg acetaminophen, 30 mg pseudoephedrine
Duragesic-25	Patch: 2.5 mg fentanyl @ 25 mcg/hour
Duragesic-50	Patch: 5 mg fentanyl @ 50 mcg/hour
Duragesic-75	Patch: 7.5 mg fentanyl @ 75 mcg/hour
Duragesic-100	Patch: 10 mg fentanyl @ 100 mcg/hour
Dura-Vent	Tablets: 75 mg phenylpropanolamine, 600 mg guaifenesin
Duridren (generic for Midrin; *see* Midrin)	
Ecotrin	Enteric Coated Tablets: 81 mg, 325 mg aspirin
Ecotrin Maximum Strength	Enteric Coated Caplets and Tablets: 500 mg aspirin
Effexor	Tablets: 25 mg, 37.5 mg, 50 mg, 75 mg, 100 mg venlafaxine
Effexor XR	Capsules: 37.5 mg, 75 mg, 150 mg venlafaxine
Elavil	Tablets: 10 mg, 25 mg, 50 mg, 75 mg, 100 mg, 150 mg amitriptyline Injection: 10 mg/ml amitriptyline
Eldepryl	Capsules: 5 mg selegiline
Entex LA	Tablets: 75 mg phenyl-propanolamine, 400 mg guaifenesin
Equagesic	Tablets: 200 mg meprobamate, 325 mg aspirin
ergonovine (*see also* Ergotrate)	Capsules: 0.2 mg (by compounding pharmacist) ergonovine
Ergotrate	Injection: 0.2 mg/ml ergonovine

Brand Name	Composition
Erythromycin Base Film Tab	Tablets: 250 mg, 500 mg erythromycin
Erythromycin Delayed Release	Capsules: 250 mg erythromycin
ephedrine (*see* Rynatuss)	
Esgic	Tablets, Capsules: 50 mg butalbital, 325 mg acetaminophen, 40 mg caffeine
Esgic Plus	Tablets: 50 mg butalbital, 500 mg acetaminophen, 40 mg caffeine
Eskalith	Capsules, Tablets: 300 mg lithium carbonate
Eskalith CR	Tablets: 450 mg lithium carbonate
Estinyl	Tablets: 0.02 mg, 0.05 mg, 0.5 mg ethinyl estrogen
Estrace	Tablets: 0.5 mg, 1 mg, 2 mg estradiol
Estraderm Transdermal System	10 cm² patch: 4 mg estradiol @ 0.05 mg/day 20 cm² patch: 8 mg estradiol @ 0.1 mg/day
estradiol (*see* Estrace, Estraderm)	
Estratab	Tablets: 0.3 mg, 0.625 mg, 1.25 mg, 2.5 mg esterified estrogens
Estratest	Tablets: 1.25 mg esterified estrogens, 2.5 mg methyltestosterone
Estratest HS	Tablets: 0.625 mg esterified estrogens, 1.25 mg methyltestosterone
ethinyl/estradiol (*see* Alesse-21, Alesse-28, Ortho-Novum 1/35, Ortho-Novum 7/7/7)	
Evista	Tablets: 60 mg raloxifene
Excedrin, Aspirin Free	Tablets, Caplets, Geltabs: 250 mg acetaminophen, 65 mg caffeine
Excedrin Extra Strength	Tablets, Caplets, Geltabs: 250 mg acetaminophen, 250 mg aspirin, 65 mg caffeine

Brand Name	Composition
Excedrin Migraine	Tablets, Caplets, Geltabs: 250 mg acetaminophen, 250 mg aspirin, 65 mg caffeine
Excedrin PM	Tablets, Caplets, Geltabs: 500 mg acetaminophen, 38 mg diphenhydramine
Fastin	Capsules: 30 mg phentermine HCl
Feldene	Capsules: 10 mg, 20 mg piroxicam
fenoprofen	Tablets: 600 mg fenoprofen calcium
fentanyl (*see* Duragesic)	
Fioricet	Tablets: 50 mg butalbital, 325 mg acetaminophen, 40 mg caffeine
Fioricet with Codeine	Capsules: 50 mg butalbital, 325 mg acetaminophen, 40 mg caffeine, 30 mg codeine
Fiorinal	Tablets, Capsules: 50 mg butalbital, 325 mg aspirin, 40 mg caffeine
Fiorinal with Codeine	Capsules: 50 mg butalbital, 325 mg aspirin, 40 mg caffeine, 30 mg codeine
Flexeril	Tablets: 10 mg cyclobenzaprine
gabapentin (*see* Neurontin)	
Glucotrol	Tablets: 5 mg, 10 mg glipizide
Glucotrol XL	Tablets: 5 mg, 10 mg glipizide
glyburide	Tablets: 1.25 mg, 2.5 mg, 5 mg glyburide
Goody's Headache Powders	Powder: aspirin, acetaminophen, caffeine
guaifenesin (*see also* Dura-Vent, Entex LA, Robitussin A-C Syrup, Ru-Tuss)	Syrup: 100 mg/5 ml guaifenesin Tablets: 600 mg guaifenesin
Halcion	Tablets: 0.125 mg, 0.25 mg triazolam
Hycodan Syrup	Syrup (per 5 ml): 5 mg hydrocodone, 1.5 mg homatropine
Hydro Diuril	Tablets: 25 mg, 50 mg, 100 mg hydrochlorothiazide

Brand Name	Composition
hydromorphone (*see* Dilaudid)	
hydroxyzine (*see also* Vistaril)	Tablets: 10 mg, 25 mg, 50 mg hydroxyzine Injection: 25 mg/ml, 50 mg/ml, 100 mg/2 ml hydroxyzine
Hygroton	Tablets: 25 mg, 50 mg chlorthalidone
hyoscyamine (*see* Cystospaz, Levsinex)	
Hytrin	Capsules: 1 mg, 2 mg, 5 mg, 10 mg terazosin
ibuprofen (*see also* Advil, Motrin IB)	Tablets: 200 mg, 400 mg, 600 mg, 800 mg ibuprofen
Imdur	Tablets: 30 mg, 60 mg, 120 mg isosorbide mononitrate
Imitrex	Tablets: 25 mg, 50 mg sumatriptan Nasal Spray: 5 mg, 20 mg sumatriptan Pre-filled Syringe Injection: 6 mg sumatriptan STAT DOSE Pre-filled Injection System: 6 mg sumatriptan Injection Vials: 6 mg/0.5 ml sumatriptan
Imuran	Tablets: 50 mg azathioprine Injection: 100 mg/20 ml azathioprine
Inderal	Tablets: 10 mg, 20 mg, 40 mg, 60 mg, 80 mg propranolol
Inderal LA	Capsules: 60 mg, 80 mg, 120 mg, 160 mg propranolol
Indocin	Capsules: 25 mg, 50 mg indomethacin Suspension: 25 mg/5 ml indomethacin Suppositories: 50 mg indomethacin
Indocin SR	Capsules: 75 mg indomethacin
Isocet (generic for Fioricet; *see* Fioricet)	
Isollyl Improved (generic for Fiorinal; *see* Fiorinal)	
Isoptin	Tablets: 40 mg, 80 mg, 120 mg verapamil

Brand Name	Composition
Isoptin SR	Tablets: 120 mg, 180 mg, 240 mg verapamil
Kadian	Capsules: 20 mg, 50 mg, 100 mg morphine sulfate
Klonopin	Tablets: 0.5 mg, 1 mg, 2 mg clonazepam
Lamictal	Tablets: 25 mg, 100 mg, 150 mg, 200 mg lamotrigine
Levsinex TimeCaps	Capsules: 0.375 hyoscyamine
Librium	Capsules: 5 mg, 10 mg, 25 mg chlordiazepoxide
Limbitrol	Tablets: 5 mg chlordiazepoxide, 12.5 mg amitriptyline
Limbitrol DS	Tablets: 10 mg chlordiazepoxide, 25 mg amitriptyline
Lipitor	Tablets: 10 mg, 20 mg, 40 mg atorvastatin calcium
lithium (*see also* Lithobid, Eskalith, Lithonate, Lithotab)	Tablets: 300 mg lithium carbonate Capsules: 150 mg, 300 mg, 600 mg lithium carbonate
Lithobid Slow Release Tabs	Tablets: 300 mg lithium carbonate
Lithonate	Capsules: 300 mg lithium carbonate
Lithotab	Tablets: 300 mg lithium carbonate
Lodine	Capsules: 200 mg, 300 mg etodolac Tablets: 400 mg, 500 mg etodolac
Lodine XL	Tablets: 400 mg, 600 mg etodolac
Loestrin Fe 1.5/30	Tablets: 1.5 mg norethindrone, 30 mcg ethinyl estradiol
Loestrin 21 1/20	Tablets: 1 mg norethindrone, 20 mcg ethinyl estradiol
Loestrin 21 1.5/30	Tablets: 1.5 mg norethindrone, 30 mcg ethinyl estradiol
Lomotil	Tablets: 2.5 mg diphenoxylate, 0.025 mg atropine sulfate Liquid (per 5 ml): 2.5 mg diphenoxylate, 0.025 atropine sulfate

Brand Name	Composition
Lo/Ovral	Tablets: 0.3 mg norgestrel, 30 mcg ethinyl estradiol
Lopressor	Tablets: 50 mg, 100 mg metoprolol tartrate Injection: 5 mg/5 ml metoprolol tartrate
Lopressor SR	Tablets: 100 mg metoprolol tartrate
Lorcet-HD	Capsules: 5 mg hydrocodone bitartrate, 500 mg acetaminophen
Lorcet Plus	Tablets: 7.5 mg hydrocodone bitartrate, 650 mg acetaminophen
Lorcet 10/650	Tablets: 10 mg hydrocodone bitartrate, 650 mg acetaminophen
Lortab ASA	Tablets: 5 mg hydrocodone bitartrate, 500 mg aspirin
Lortab Elixir	Liquid (per 15 ml): 7.5 mg hydrocodone bitartrate, 500 mg acetaminophen
Lortab 2.5/500	Tablets: 2.5 mg hydrocodone bitartrate, 500 mg acetaminophen
Lortab 5/500	Tablets: 5 mg hydrocodone bitartrate, 500 mg acetaminophen
Lortab 7.5/500	Tablets: 7.5 mg hydrocodone bitartrate, 500 mg acetaminophen
Lortab 10/500	Tablets: 10 mg hydrocodone bitartrate, 500 mg acetaminophen
lovastatin (*see* Mevacor)	
Lupron Depot 3.75 mg	Suspension for injection: 3.75 mg leuprolide acetate
Lupron Depot 7.5 mg	Suspension for injection: 7.5 mg leuprolide acetate
Lupron Depot-3 month 11.25 mg	Suspension for injection: 11.25 mg leuprolide acetate
Lupron Depot-3 month 22.5 mg	Suspension for injection: 22.5 mg leuprolide acetate
Lupron Depot-4 month 30 mg	Suspension for injection: 30 mg leuprolide acetate

Brand Name	Composition
Luvox	Tablets: 25 mg, 50 mg, 100 mg fluvoxamine maleate
Macrodantin	Capsules: 25 mg, 50 mg, 100 mg nitrofurantoin macrocrystals
magnesium oxide (*see also* Mag-Ox 400)	Tablets: 250 mg magnesium oxide (OTC)
Mag-Ox 400	Tablets: 400 mg magnesium oxide
Maxalt	Tablets: 5 mg, 10 mg rizatriptan
Maxalt MLT	Orally disintegrating tablets: 5 mg, 10 mg rizatriptan
meclizine (*see* Antivert)	
Medrol (*see also* Depo-Medrol)	Tablets: 2 mg, 4 mg, 6 mg, 8 mg, 16 mg, 24 mg, 32 mg methylprednisolone
	Injection: 20 mg/ml, 40 mg/ml, 80 mg/ml methylprednisolone acetate
medroxyprogesterone acetate (*see* Premphase, Prempro, Provera)	
Mellaril	Tablets: 10 mg, 15 mg, 25 mg, 50 mg, 100 mg, 150 mg, 200 mg thioridazine
Meridia	Capsules: 5 mg, 10 mg, 15 mg sibutramine
methadone (Dolophine)	Tablets: 5 mg, 10 mg methadone
	Injection: 10 mg/ml methadone
metoclopramide (*see* Reglan)	
methylphenidate (*see* Ritalin)	
Mevacor	Tablets: 10 mg, 20 mg, 40 mg lovastatin
Micronor	Tablets: 0.35 mg norethindrone
Midol-200	Tablets: 200 mg ibuprofen
Midol Maximum Strength Multi-Symptom	Caplets: 500 mg acetaminophen, 15 mg pyrilamine maleate, 60 mg caffeine
Midol PMS Multi-Symptom	Caplets: 500 mg acetaminophen, 25 mg pamabrom, 15 mg pyrilamine maleate

Brand Name	Composition
Midol Teen	Caplets: 500 mg acetaminophen, 25 mg pamabrom
Midrin	Capsules: 65 mg isometheptene mucate, 100 mg dichlo-ralphenazone, 325 mg acetaminophen
Migranal Nasal Spray	Nasal Spray: 4 mg/ml dihydroergotamine mesylate @ 0.5 mg per spray
Moduretic	Tablets: 5 mg amiloride, 50 mg hydrochlorothiazide
morphine (*see* Kadian, MS Contin)	
Motrin	Tablets: 300 mg, 400 mg, 600 mg, 800 mg ibuprofen
Motrin, Children's	Drops: 50 mg/1.25 ml ibuprofen Suspension: 100 mg/5 ml ibuprofen Chewable tablets: 50 mg ibuprofen
Motrin IB	Tablets, Caplets, Gelcaps: 200 mg ibuprofen
Motrin IB Sinus	Tablets, Caplets: 200 mg ibuprofen, 30 mg pseudoephedrine
Motrin Junior Strength	Chewable Tablets, Caplets: 100 mg ibuprofen
MS Contin Controlled Release Tabs	Tablets: 15 mg, 30 mg, 60 mg, 100 mg morphine sulfate
Naprelan	Tablets: 375 mg, 500 mg naproxen sodium
Naprosyn	Tablets: 250 mg, 375 mg, 500 mg naproxen Suspension: 125 mg/5 ml naproxen
Naprosyn, EC Delayed Release Tabs	Tablets: 375 mg, 500 mg naproxen
Nardil	Tablets: 15 mg phenelzine sulfate
nefazodone (*see* Serzone)	
Neurontin	Capsules: 100 mg, 300 mg, 400 mg gabapentin
Nimotop	Capsules: 30 mg nimodipine
Nolvadex	Tablets: 10 mg, 20 mg tamoxifen citrate

Brand Name	Composition
Norflex	Tablets: 100 mg orphenadrine citrate Injection: 30 mg/ml orphenadrine citrate
Norgesic	Tablets: 25 mg orphenadrine citrate, 385 mg aspirin, 30 mg caffeine
Norgesic Forte	Tablets: 50 mg orphenadrine citrate, 770 mg aspirin, 60 mg caffeine
Norpramin	Tablets: 10 mg, 25 mg, 50 mg, 75 mg, 100 mg, 150 mg desipramine
nortriptyline (*see* Pamelor, Aventyl)	
Nubain	Injection: 10 mg/ml, 20 mg/ml nalbuphine
Nuprin	Tablets, Caplets: 200 mg ibuprofen
Ortho-Novum 1/35 (21 and 28 tablet packs)	Tablets: 1 mg norethindrone, 35 mcg ethinyl estradiol
Ortho-Novum 7/7/7 (21 and 28 tablet packs)	Phase I Tablets: 0.5 mg norethindrone, 35 mcg ethinyl estradiol Phase II Tablets: 0.75 mg norethindrone, 35 mcg ethinyl estradiol Phase III Tablets: 1 mg norethindrone, 35 mcg ethinyl estradiol
Orudis	Capsules: 25 mg, 50 mg, 75 mg ketoprofen
OrudisKT	Tablets: 12.5 mg ketoprofen
Oruvail	Capsules: 100 mg, 150 mg, 200 mg ketoprofen
oxycodone (*see* Oxycontin, Percocet, Percodan, Roxicet)	
Oxycontin	Tablets: 10 mg, 20 mg, 40 mg oxycodone
Pamelor	Capsules: 10 mg, 25 mg, 50 mg, 75 mg nortriptyline
Pamprin Multi-Symptom	Tablets: 500 mg acetaminophen, 25 mg pamabrom, 15 mg pyrilamine
Parafon Forte DSC	Caplets: 500 mg chlorzoxazone

Brand Name	Composition
Parlodel	Snap Tabs: 2.5 mg bromocriptine mesylate Capsules: 5 mg bromocriptine mesylate
Paxil	Tablets: 10 mg, 20 mg, 30 mg, 40 mg paroxetine
Pepcid	Tablets: 20 mg, 40 mg famotidine Suspension: 40 mg/5 ml famotidine Injection: 10 mg/ml famotidine
Pepcid AC	Tablets: 10 mg famotidine
Percocet	Tablets: 5 mg oxycodone, 325 mg acetaminophen
Percodan	Tablets: 4.5 mg oxycodone, 0.38 mg oxycodone terephthalate, 325 mg aspirin
Percodan-Demi	Tablets: 2.25 mg oxycodone, 0.19 mg oxycodone terephthalate, 325 mg aspirin
Percogesic	Tablets: 30 mg phenyltoloxamine citrate, 325 mg acetaminophen
Periactin	Tablets: 4 mg cyproheptadine Syrup: 2 mg/5 ml cyproheptadine
Phenergan	Tablets: 12.5 mg, 25 mg, 50 mg promethazine Suppositories: 12.5 mg, 25 mg, 50 mg promethazine
Phenergan Fortis Syrup	Syrup: 25 mg/5 ml promethazine
Phenergan Plain Syrup	Syrup: 6.25 mg/5 ml promethazine
Phenergan VC Syrup	Syrup (per 5 ml): 6.25 mg promethazine, 5 mg phenylephrine
Phenergan VC with Codeine Syrup	Syrup (per 5 ml): 6.25 mg promethazine, 5 mg phenylephrine, 10 mg codeine
Phenergan with Codeine Syrup	Syrup (per 5 ml): 6.25 mg promethazine, 10 mg codeine
phentermine (*see also* Adipex-P, Fastin)	Capsules: 15 mg, 30 mg, 37.5 mg phentermine
Phrenilin	Tablets: 50 mg butalbital, 325 mg acetaminophen

Brand Name	Composition
Phrenilin Forte	Capsules: 50 mg butalbital, 650 mg acetaminophen
Pravachol	Tablets: 10 mg, 20 mg, 40 mg pravastatin sodium
prednisone	Tablets: 1 mg, 2.5 mg, 5 mg, 10 mg, 20 mg, 50 mg prednisone Oral Solution: 5 mg/5 ml prednisone
Premarin	Tablets: 0.3 mg, 0.625 mg, 0.9 mg, 1.25 mg, 2.5 mg conjugated estrogens
Premphase	Phase I Tablets: 0.625 mg conjugated estrogens Phase II Tablets: 0.625 mg conjugated estrogens, 5 mg medroxyprogesterone acetate
Prempro	Tablets: 0.625 mg conjugated estrogens, 2.5 mg medroxy-progesterone acetate
Prevacid	Capsules: 15 mg, 30 mg lansoprazole
Prilosec	Capsules: 10 mg, 20 mg, 40 mg omeprazole
progesterone (*see also* Provera, Premphase, Prempro)	Tablets: 2.5 mg, 5 mg, 10 mg medroxyprogesterone acetate
Procardia	Capsules: 10 mg, 20 mg nifedipine
Procardia XL	Tablets: 30 mg, 60 mg, 90 mg nifedipine
Provera	Tablets: 2.5 mg, 5 mg, 10 mg medroxyprogesterone acetate
Prozac	Pulvules: 10 mg, 20 mg fluoxetine Liquid: 20 mg/5ml fluoxetine
raloxifene (*see* Evista)	
Reglan	Tablets: 5 mg, 10 mg metoclopramide Syrup: 5 mg/5 ml metoclopramide Injection: 5 mg/5 ml metoclopramide
Remeron	Tablets: 15 mg, 30 mg mirtazapine
Risperdal	Tablets: 1 mg, 2 mg, 3 mg, 4 mg risperidone

Brand Name	Composition
Ritalin	Tablets: 5 mg, 10 mg, 20 mg methylphenidate
Ritalin SR	Tablets: 20 mg methylphenidate
Robaxin	Tablets: 500 mg methocarbamol Injection: 100 mg/ml methocarbamol
Robaxin-750	Tablets: 750 mg methocarbamol
Robitussin A-C Syrup	Syrup (per 5 ml): 100 mg guaifenesin, 10 mg codeine, 3.5% alcohol
Roxicet	Tablets: 5 mg oxycodone, 325 mg acetaminophen Oral solution (per 5 ml): 5 mg oxycodone, 325 mg acetaminophen
Roxicet 5/500	Caplets: 5 mg oxycodone, 500 mg acetaminophen
Roxanol, Roxanol-T	Oral solution: 20 mg/ml morphine sulfate
Roxanal 100	Oral solution: 100 mg/5 ml morphine sulfate
Ru-Tuss	Tablets: 25 mg phenylephrine, 50 mg phenylpropanolamine, 8 mg chlorpheniramine, 0.19 mg hyoscyamine, 0.04 mg atropine, 0.01 scopolamine
Rynatuss	Tablets: 60 mg carbetapentane tannate, 5 mg chlorpheniramine tannate, 10 mg ephedrine tannate, 10 mg phenylephrine tannate Suspension (per 5 ml): 30 mg carbetapentane tannate, 4 mg chlorpheniramine tannate, 5 mg ephedrine tannate, 5 mg phenylephrine tannate
Sansert	Tablets: 2 mg methysergide
Serax	Capsules: 10 mg, 15 mg, 30 mg oxazepam Tablets: 15 mg oxazepam
Seroquel	Tablets: 25 mg, 100 mg, 200 mg quetiapine

Brand Name	Composition
Serzone	Tablets: 100 mg, 150 mg, 200 mg, 250 mg nefazodone
Sine-Aid IB	Tablets, Caplets: 200 mg ibuprofen, 30 mg pseudoephedrine
Sine-Aid Maximum Strength	Tablets, Caplets: 500 mg acetaminophen, 30 mg pseudoephedrine
Sine-Off	Tablets: 30 mg pseudoephedrine, 2 mg chlorpheniramine, 500 mg acetaminophen
Sinequan	Capsules: 10 mg, 25 mg, 50 mg, 75 mg, 100 mg, 150 mg doxepin Oral concentrate: 10 mg/ml doxepin
Singulair	5 mg, 10 mg montelukast
Sinutab Maximum Strength Sinus Allergy	Tablets: 500 mg acetaminophen, 2 mg chlorpheniramine, 30 mg pseudoephedrine
Skelaxin	Tablets: 400 mg metaxalone
Soma	Tablets: 350 mg carisoprodol
Soma Compound	Tablets: 200 mg carisoprodol, 325 mg aspirin
Sonata	Tablets: 5 mg, 10 mg zaleplon
Stadol	Injection: 1 mg/ml, 2 mg/ml butorphanol
Stadol Nasal Spray	Nasal Spray: 10 mg/ml butorphanol @ 1 mg per spray
St. Joseph's Adult Chewable Aspirin	Tablet: 81 mg aspirin
Sudafed	Tablets: 30 mg pseudoephedrine
Sudafed 12-Hour	Caplets: 120 mg pseudoephedrine
Sudafed Plus	Tablets, Caplets: 60 mg pseudoephedrine, 4 mg chlorpheniramine
Sudafed Sinus	Tablets, Caplets: 30 mg pseudoephedrine, 500 mg acetaminophen
Surmontil	Capsules: 25 mg, 50 mg, 100 mg trimipramine maleate

Brand Name	Composition
Synalgos-DC	Capsules: 16 mg dihydrocodeine bitartrate, 356.4 mg aspirin, 30 mg caffeine
Synthroid	Tablets: 25 mcg, 50 mcg, 75 mcg, 88 mcg, 100 mcg, 112 mcg, 125 mcg, 150 mcg, 175 mcg, 200 mcg, 300 mcg levothyroxine sodium Injection: 200 mcg/10 ml, 500 mcg/10 ml levothyroxine sodium
Tagamet	Tablets: 200 mg, 300 mg, 400 mg, 800 mg cimetidine
Tagamet HB	Tablets: 200 mg cimetidine
Talacen	Caplets: 25 mg pentazocine, 650 mg acetaminophen
Talwin Compound	Caplets: 12.5 mg pentazocine, 325 mg aspirin
Talwin Nx	Tablets: 50 mg pentazocine, 0.5 mg naloxone
Tavist D	Tablets: 1.34 mg clemastine, 75 mg phenylpropanolamine
Tavist Sinus	Tablets: 500 mg acetaminophen, 30 mg pseudoephedrine
Tegretol	Chewable tablets: 100 mg, 200 mg carbamazepine Tablets: 200 mg carbamazepine
Tegretol CR	Capsules: 200 mg, 400 mg carbamazepine
Tegretol XR	Tablets: 100 mg, 200 mg, 400 mg carbamazepine
Tenormin	Tablets: 25 mg, 50 mg, 100 mg atenolol
Testoderm Transdermal System	Patch: 4 mg/day, 6 mg/day testosterone
Testoderm Transdermal System with Adhesive	Patch: 6 mg/day testosterone
testosterone (*see* Androderm, Testoderm)	

Brand Name	Composition
Thorazine	Tablets: 10 mg, 25 mg, 50 mg, 100 mg, 200 mg chlorpromazine Spansule: 30 mg, 75 mg, 150 mg chlorpromazine Suppositories: 25 mg, 100 mg chlorpromazine Syrup: 10 mg/5 ml chlorpromazine Injection: 25 mg/ml chlorpromazine
Tigan	Capsules: 100 mg, 250 mg trimethobenzamide Suppositories: 100 mg, 200 mg trimethobenzamide Injection: 100 mg/ml trimethobenzamide
Tofranil-PM	Capsules: 75 mg, 100 mg, 125 mg, 150 mg imipramine pamoate
Topamax	Tablets: 25 mg, 100 mg, 200 mg topiramate
Toradol	IV/IM Tubex, IV/IM Sterile Vials: 15 mg/ml, 30 mg/ml ketorolac IM Tubex One-time Use: 60 mg/ 2 ml ketorolac tromethamine IV Tubex Blunt Pointe: 15 mg/ml, 30 mg/ml ketorolac tromethamine Tablets: 10 mg ketorolac tromethamine
Tranxene	Tablets: 3.75 mg, 7.5 mg, 15 mg clorazepate dipotassium
Tranxene SD	Tablets: 22.5 mg clorazepate dipotassium
Tranxene SD Half Strength	Tablets: 11.25 mg clorazepate dipotassium
Triaminic Cold	Tablets: 12.5 mg phenylpropanolamine, 2 mg chlorpheniramine
Trileptal	Tablets: 150 mg, 300 mg, 600 mg oxcarbazepine
Tylenol, Children's	Chewable tablets: 80 mg acetaminophen Elixir, Suspension: 160 mg/ 5 ml acetaminophen

Brand Name	Composition
Tylenol Allergy-D, Children's	Liquid (per 5 ml): 160 mg acetaminophen, 12.5 mg diphenhydramine, 15 mg pseudoephedrine
Tylenol Cold, Children's	Chewable tablets: 80 mg acetaminophen, 0.5 mg chlorpheniramine maleate, 7.5 mg pseudoephedrine Liquid (per 5 ml): 160 mg acetaminophen, 1 mg chlorpheniramine maleate, 15 mg pseudoephedrine
Tylenol Flu, Children's	Liquid (per 5 ml): 160 mg acetaminophen, 7.5 mg diphenhydramine, 15 mg pseudoephedrine, 1 mg chlorpheniramine
Tylenol Cold Medication No Drowsiness Formula	Caplets, Gelcaps: 325 mg acetaminophen, 15 mg dextromethorphan, 30 mg pseudoephedrine
Tylenol Cold Multi-Symptom	Tablets, Caplets: 325 mg acetaminophen, 15 mg dextromethorphan, 30 mg pseudoephedrine, 2 mg chlorpheniramine
Tylenol, Extended Relief	Caplets: 650 mg acetaminophen
Tylenol, Extra Strength	Tablets, Caplets, Gelcaps, Geltabs: 500 mg acetaminophen
Tylenol PM, Extra Strength	Tablets, Caplets, Gelcaps: 500 mg acetaminophen, 25 mg diphenhydramine
Tylenol Maximum Strength Allergy Sinus	Caplets, Gelcaps: 500 mg acetaminophen, 2 mg chlorpheniramine, 30 mg pseudoephedrine
Tylenol, Regular Strength	Caplets, Tablets: 325 mg acetaminophen
Tylenol Severe Allergy	Caplets: 500 mg acetaminophen, 12.5 mg diphenhydramine
Tylenol with Codeine #3	Tablets: 30 mg codeine, 300 mg acetaminophen

Brand Name	Composition
Tylenol with Codeine #4	Tablets: 60 mg codeine, 300 mg acetaminophen
Tylox	Capsules: 5 mg oxycodone, 500 mg acetaminophen
Ultram	Tablets: 50 mg tramadol
Valium	Tablets: 2 mg, 5 mg, 10 mg diazepam
Vanquish	Tablets: 227 mg aspirin, 194 mg acetaminophen, 33 mg caffeine
Vasotec	Tablets: 2.5 mg, 5 mg, 10 mg, 20 mg enalapril maleate
verapamil (*see* Calan, Calan SR, Covera HS, Isoptin, Isoptin SR)	
Vicodin	Tablets: 5 mg hydrocodone, 500 mg acetaminophen
Vicodin ES	Tablets: 7.5 mg hydrocodone, 750 mg acetaminophen
Vicodin HP	Tablets: 10 mg hydrocodone, 660 mg acetaminophen
Vicoprofen	Tablets: 7.5 mg hydrocodone, 200 mg ibuprofen
Vistaril	Capsules: 25 mg, 50 mg, 100 mg hydroxyzine pamoate
Vivactil	Tablets: 5 mg, 10 mg protriptyline
Voltaren	Tablets: 25 mg, 50 mg, 75 mg diclofenac sodium
Voltaren XR	Tablets: 100 mg diclofenac sodium
Wellbutrin	Tablets: 75 mg bupropion
Wellbutrin SR	Tablets: 100 mg, 150 mg bupropion
Wigraine	Tablets: 1 mg ergotamine tartrate, 100 mg caffeine Suppositories: 2 mg ergotamine tartrate, 100 mg caffeine
Xanax	Tablets: 0.25 mg, 0.5 mg, 1 mg, 2 mg alprazolam

Brand Name	Composition
Zantac	Efferdose Tabs, Granules: 150 mg ranitidine Tablets, Capsules: 150 mg, 300 mg ranitidine
Zantac 75	Tablets: 75 mg ranitidine
Ziac 6.25/2.5	Tablets: 6.25 mg hydrochlorothiazide, 2.5 mg bisoprolol fumarate
Ziac 6.25/5	Tablets: 6.25 mg hydrochlorothiazide, 5 mg bisoprolol fumarate
Ziac 6.25/10	Tablets: 6.25 mg hydrochlorothiazide, 10 mg bisoprolol fumarate
Zithromax	Tablets: 250 mg, 600 mg azithromycin Capsules: 250 mg azithromycin Suspension (per bottle): 300 mg, 600 mg, 900 mg, 1200 mg azithromycin @ 100 mg/5 ml, 200 mg/5 ml Suspension (Single Dose Packets): 1000 mg azithromycin dihydrate
Zocor	Tablets: 5 mg, 10 mg, 20 mg, 40 mg simvastatin
Zofran	Tablets: 4 mg, 8 mg ondansetron dihydrate Oral solution: 4 mg/5 ml ondansetron
Zofran ODT	Orally disintegrating tablets: 4 mg, 8 mg
Zoloft	Tablets: 25 mg, 50 mg, 100 mg sertraline
zolpidem (*see* Ambien)	
Zomig	Tablets: 2.5 mg, 5 mg zolmitriptan
Zyprexa	Tablets: 2.5 mg, 5 mg, 7.5 mg, 10 mg, 15 mg olanzapine

ACKNOWLEDGMENTS

· · · · · · · · · · · · · · · · ·

I would like to first thank my coauthor, Susan, and our editor, Rux Martin. I want to thank my wife, Suzy, for her continuing love and support, and my dad, Joseph, for a lifetime of caring. I am grateful to my wonderful son, Michael, and stepchildren, Daniel and Carly, for adding meaning to my life. And thank you to Dorrie, Karen W., Phyllis, Karen S., and Dr. L., for improving the quality of life for our patients.

— L.D.R.

First I want to thank Larry Bernard of the Cornell News Service for connecting me with my coauthor. I want to thank my dad, Solon J. Lang, for his love, intellectual guidance, and support over the years. And I want to thank my husband, Tom Schneider, and my daughter, Julia Lang Schneider, for their continuing love and support.

— S.S.L.

INDEX

· · · · · ·

Abortive medications, 9; for adolescents' headaches, 208–9; for children's headaches, 198–203; for cluster headaches, 175–78; for migraines, 63, 64, 65–77, 91, 127, 230; for tension headaches, 145–51

Academy for Guided Imagery, 269

Acceptance, 41

Acetaminophen, 8, 19, 29, 32–33, 137, 138, 145, 146, 195, 196–97, 209, 210, 239, 282–90

Acetaminophen with codeine, 82, 137

Aciphex, 39

Aconite, 254

Actifed, 287, 291

Acupressure, 257

Acupressure Institute, 275

Acupuncture, 255–57, 275–76

Adderall, 291

Addiction, 77–78, 84; to abortive medications, 9; to butalbital compounds, 65, 75; to cocaine, 185; vs. dependency, 77, 149, 263; to methylphenidate, 186; to narcotics, 81–82, 174, 177; to stimulants, 124; and tension-headache medications, 148–49

Adipex-P, 291

Adolescents' headaches, 207–15; case study on, 218–20; counseling for, 194. See also Children's headaches

Advil, 8, 19, 31, 72, 146, 147, 157, 195, 197, 286, 287, 291

After-surgery headaches, 239

Alcohol, 40, 98, 99, 131, 173, 219, 237, 239–40, 264

Aldactone, 291

Alesse-21/28, 292

Aleve, 31, 71, 105, 114–15, 145, 147, 157, 177, 195, 199, 209, 210, 211, 219, 286, 292; and Cox-2 inhibitor, 72. See also Naproxen

Alka-Seltzer, 286, 292

Allerest, 292

Allergy headaches, 15, 235–36

Allergy-Sinus Comtrex, 289

Altace, 292

Alternative headache treatments, 246–64. See also Self-help strategies

Alternative medicine organizations, 274–75

Altitude, and migraines, 102

Ambien, 292

Amerge, 292; for children's and adolescents' headaches, 196, 203, 211; for cluster headaches, 175, 183; for exertional headaches, 232; and MAO inhibitors, 122; for migraines, 64, 65, 67, 70, 119, 121, 125, 131, 132, 136, 139; for post-traumatic migraines, 231; for tension headaches, 150, 151

American Academy of Medical Acupuncture, 256, 276

American Academy of Osteopathy, 277

American Association of Acupuncture and Oriental Medicine, 276

American Association of Naturopathic Physicians, 275

American Botanical Council, 273

American Chiropractic Association, 279–80

American Chronic Pain Association, 274

American Council for Headache Education (ACHE), 267–68

American Foundation of Traditional Chinese Medicine, 276

American Herb Association, 272

American Holistic Medical Association, 275

American Institute of Hypnotherapy, 277

American Massage Therapy Association, 277

American Oriental Bodywork Association, 276

American Osteopathic Association, 277

American Psychiatric Association, 270

American Psychological Association, 270

American Self-Help Clearinghouse, 268

American Sleep Disorders Association, 278

American Society for Clinical Hypnosis, 277–78

Amitriptyline: for adolescents' headaches, 213; and beta-blockers, 112; for children's headaches, 206, 207; for cluster headaches, 186; headaches caused by, 242; and hemicrania continua, 240; for migraines, 106–7, 111, 137; with naproxen, 118; for older people's headaches, 223, 224, 225; for post-traumatic headaches, 230; with propranolol, 118, 161; for tension headaches, 154. *See also* Antidepressants

Amphetamines, 121, 161, 162–63

Anacin, 32, 65, 73, 146, 147, 210, 284, 292; Aspirin Free, 282, 292; caffeine in, 28, 284

Analgesics, 233, 235, 242. *See also* Acetaminophen; Aspirin

Anaprox, 31, 105, 114–15, 157, 195, 199, 210, 292. *See also* Naproxen

Anaprox DS, 145, 177, 292

Androderm Transdermal System, 292

Anemia, and headaches, 56

Anodynos, 30

Ansaid, 105, 115, 157, 232, 292. *See also* Flurbiprofen

Antacids, 86, 87–88

Antibiotics, 242

Antidepressants: for adolescents' headaches, 213, 214; and back-of-the-head pain, 241; and breastfeeding, 138; for children's headaches, 205, 206–7; for cluster headaches, 186; Depakote with, 118, 161; headaches caused by, 242; for migraines, 104, 106–12, 144; for older people's headaches, 223, 224, 225; for post-traumatic headaches, 230–31; and St.-John's-Wort, 249; and serotonin, 6; and tension headaches, 144, 153, 154–56

Antiemetics, 69

Antihistamines, 138, 235

Anti-inflammatories, 144, 174, 212, 213, 214, 221, 222, 223, 227, 230, 231, 232, 241; with beta-blockers, 159; headaches caused by, 242

Anti-inflammatories, nonsteroidal. *See* Nonsteroidal anti-inflammatories

Antinausea medications: brand-name, 290; and breastfeeding, 138; for children, 199, 203–4; for cluster headaches, 174, 175, 178; for migraines, 63, 69, 73, 86, 87–90, 131, 137; and narcotics, 79

Antivert, 292

Anxiety, 58, 96, 105, 107, 112, 207–8, 262

Anxiety Disorder Education Program/ National Institute of Mental Health, 271

Anxiety Disorders Association of America, 270–71

Aristocort, 180

Aromatherapy, 253, 273–74

Aromatherapy Quarterly, 274

Arrestin, 89

Arteritis, temporal, 226–27

Arthritis, 56, 72, 156, 221, 227

Arthritis Pain Formula, 284, 293

Arthritis Strength Anacin Tablets, 284

Arthritis Strength Bufferin, 285

Arthrotec, 293

Ascriptin, 284–85, 286

Aspartame, 99

Aspergum, 201, 284

Aspirin, 19, 29, 32, 282–90; for after-surgery headaches, 239; for children or adolescents, 196, 201–2, 209, 210, 211; and Cox-2 inhibitor, 72; and feverfew, 248; headaches caused by, 242; for migraines, 65, 70; and nausea, 30; for post-traumatic headaches, 230; and rebound headaches, 8; stomach problems from, 39; for tension headaches, 145, 147, 157. *See also* Nonsteroidal anti-inflammatories

Aspirin with codeine, 82

Aspirin Free Anacin, 282, 292

Aspirin Free Excedrin, 31–32, 73, 146, 196–97, 210, 282, 300

Assessment Form, 45, 52–54

Association for Advancement of Behavior Therapy (AABT), 270

Association for Applied Psychophysiology and Biofeedback, 269

Asthma, 112, 113, 126, 262

Atenolol, 113, 242. *See also* Beta-blockers
Athletics, and calcium blockers, 116
Ativan, 293
Attention deficit disorder (ADD), organization for, 279
Auras, 12, 45, 57, 58, 59–60, 61, 62, 192
Autogenic training, 24–25
Aventyl, 109, 111, 155, 206, 213, 293. *See also* Nortriptyline
Axid, 39, 293
Axocet, 293

Bancap HC, 293
Baths, 27
Bayer Aspirin, 211, 284, 285, 293
Bayer Children's Chewable Aspirin, 283, 293
Bayer Enteric Aspirin, 293
Bayer Select Ibuprofen Pain Relief Formula, 286
BC Arthritis Strength, 286
BC Headache Powders, 30, 65, 73, 284, 285, 293
BC Tablets, 30, 286
Belcomp, 294
Belladonna, 254
Bellergal-S, 179, 182, 183. *See also* Ergotamine(s)
Belleruth Naparstek, Image Paths, Inc., 269
Benadryl, 289, 293
Benson, Herbert, 21
Bentyl, 294
Benzacot, 89
Benzodiazepines, 84, 148–49, 149, 151, 222. *See also* Sedatives
Beta-blockers: for adolescents, 214; and asthma, 126; and breastfeeding, 138; for cluster headaches, 186; in combination, 161; for migraines, 105, 112–14, 137, 144; for older people's headaches, 223, 224; for post-traumatic headaches, 230; and tension headaches, 144, 158–59
Betamethasone, 184. *See also* Cortisone
Biofeedback, 26–27, 194, 230, 255; organizations on, 269–70
Bio-Gan, 89
Biotene toothpaste, 107
Bipolar illness (manic-depression), 106
Bipuvacaine, 168
Birth control pills, 101, 129, 132, 135–36

Blocadren, 113–14, 294. *See also* Timolol
Blood tests, 48
Blood thinners, and feverfew, 248
Blue Poppy Press, 276
Botulinum (Botox) injections, 187, 254, 260–61
Brain, and headaches, 4, 5, 47, 56, 129, 171–72, 221, 251, 279
Brain Injury Association, 279
Brain tumors, 12, 47, 244, 280
Breastfeeding, headache during, 138. *See also* Nursing women
Breathing exercises, 19–27, 263
Bright lights, 35, 101
Bromocriptine. *See* Parlodel
Bromo-Seltzer, 28, 294
Bruxism, 236
Bryonia, 254
Bufferin, 285, 294
Buffets II, 30
Bumex, 294
Bupropion, 110, 111
Burns, David D., 36
Buspar, 294
Butalbital compounds, 65, 75–77, 148, 149, 150, 177, 196, 200–201, 211, 222
Butorphanol, 83. *See also* Stadol Nasal Spray

Cafergot, 70, 78, 79–80, 179, 182, 183, 222, 294. *See also* Ergotamine(s)
Cafergot PB, 80, 294
Caffeine, 3, 10, 19, 27–29, 282–90; for adolescents' headaches, 210; and breastfeeding, 138; for children's headaches, 195, 196, 198; in feverfew, 248; and gastrointestinal tract, 39; in guarana, 250; with ibuprofen, 31; with ketoprofen, 148; and MAO inhibitors, 122; and migraines, 63, 65, 98, 131; and older people, 222; and pregnancy, 137; and rebound headaches, 8, 29, 98, 146, 147, 242; and sinus headaches, 235; and sleep, 40; and spinal tap headaches, 233; for tension headaches, 146, 147; and weekend headaches, 29, 96, 238
Caffeine-aspirin combinations, 146, 147
Calan, 105, 116, 158, 160, 181, 214, 294. *See also* Verapamil
Calan SR, 294

Calcium, 136, 252

Calcium blockers: headaches caused by, 15, 242; and hemicrania continua, 240; for migraines, 105, 115–16; for post-traumatic headaches, 231; for tension headaches, 138, 139, 144, 158, 160, 161

Calendar, as headache record, 34–35, 42–43, 45, 94

Calm-X, 88

Cancer, 244

Captropril, 242

Carbamazepine, 241

Cardizem, 116, 294

Cardizem CD, 294

Cardizem SR, 294

Carotid artery, and headaches, 172

Case studies: on children's and adolescents' headaches, 215–20; on cluster headaches, 187–90; on migraines, 90–93, 125–28, 140–41, 215–20; on tension headaches, 163–70

Cataflam, 105

Catapres, 295

Catapres Transdermal Therapeutic Systems, 295

CAT (computerized axial tomography) scan, 47

Celebrex, 64, 71, 72, 105, 114, 115, 156, 221–22, 222, 295. *See also* Nonsteroidal anti-inflammatories

Celexa, 15, 111, 139, 231, 295

Center for Alternative Medicine Clearinghouse, 275

Center for Mind-Body Medicine, 275

Cervicogenic headache, 241

Chamomile, 41, 247, 249, 253

Cheeses, 98, 122, 131, 173

Children and Adults with Attention Deficit Disorders (CHADD), 279

Children's headaches, 191–92; and antinausea medications, 199, 203–4; case studies on, 215–18; medications for, 195–203, 205–7; nondrug strategies for, 191, 193–94; and stress, 217; symptoms of, 192–93. *See also* Adolescents' headaches

Chinese medicine, organization on, 276

Chiropractic therapy, 38, 258, 279–80

Chlordiazepoxide, 149, 151, 162. *See also* Sedatives; Tranquilizers

Chlorpromazine, 87, 89, 178. *See also* Antinausea medications

Chlor-Trimeton, 287

Chocolate, 98, 122, 131, 173, 235

Chronic pain, organizations for, 274

Chronic paroxysmal hemicrania (CPH), 184, 240, 241

Cigarette smoke. *See* Smoke; Smoking

Cimetidine, 39, 242. *See also* Tagamet

Circulatory problems, headaches caused by, 243–44

Citalopram, 111. *See also* Celexa

Claritin, 295

Claritin-D, 295

Clonazepam, 84, 149, 151, 162

Cluster headaches, 13, 14, 171–73; after age fifty, 221, 225–26; and blood pressure, 244; case studies on, 187–90; and chronic paroxysmal hemicrania, 240; gamma knife radiation for, 187; medications for, 174–86; and migraine symptoms, 59; nondrug strategies for, 173–74; surgery for, 186–87; trigger-point injections for, 254

Cocaine, 242

Cocaine solution, 180, 185

Codeine, 69, 78, 82, 137, 149, 150, 222. *See also* Narcotics

Coffee, 28, 39. *See also* Caffeine

Cold, as nondrug therapy, 33

Cold preparations, 242

Compazine, 69, 86, 87, 88, 131, 137, 138, 178, 203, 295

Comtrex, 288, 289, 295

Contac, 295

Cool dark room, as self-help, 34

Cope, 28, 30, 286

Coping skills, 36–37

Corgard, 105, 113, 158, 159, 186, 230, 295

Coronary artery disease (CAD), after age fifty, 225–26

Corticosteroids, 78, 81

Cortisone, 92, 137, 178, 179, 180–81, 184, 235, 241, 254

Cough headaches, 232

Coumadin, and feverfew, 248

Counseling, 194, 208, 230, 270–72

Covera HS, 181, 295

Cox-2 inhibitors, 72, 114, 115, 157, 221–22, 222, 224

Cozaar, 295

Cranial Academy, The, 277

Craniosacral therapy, organizations on, 277

Crinone, 296

Cyclobenzaprine, 159–60, 230

Cylert, 296

Cyproheptadine. *See* Periactin

Cystospaz, 296

Cystospaz-M, 296

Cytomel, 296

Dallergy, 296

Dalmane, 296

Danazol, 242

Darvocet, 82, 149, 150, 163

Darvocet N-100, 296

Darvon, 78, 82, 149, 150, 296

Darvon Compound-65, 296

Darvon N, 296

Daypro, 296

Decadron, 78, 81, 92, 131, 180, 202, 261, 296

Deltasone, 296

Demerol, 78, 83, 122, 137, 296

Demulen 1/50, 296

Depacon, 261, 296. *See also* Valproate

Depakote, 104, 105–6, 138, 153, 154, 296; for adolescents' headaches, 213, 214; for cluster headaches, 179, 182; in combination, 118, 161; for older people's headaches, 223, 224; for post-traumatic headaches, 230

Dependence, vs. addiction, 77, 149, 263

Depo-Medrol, 78, 81, 180, 184, 261, 296. *See also* Cortisone

Depression: and adolescents' headaches, 207–8; and Depakote, 105; and headaches after age fifty, 221; and kava kava, 249; and magnet therapy, 260; as migraine trigger, 96; and St.-John's-Wort, 249; from serotonin lack, 262

Depression Awareness Recognition and Treatment Education Program (DART), 272

Depression and Related Affective Disorders Association (DRADA), 271

Desipramine, 110, 111, 155. *See also* Norpramin

Desyrel, 297

Dexamethasone, 81, 92, 180. *See also* Decadron

Dexedrine, 161, 163, 297

Dextroamphetamine, 121, 124, 163, 263

DHE (dihydroergotamine), 6, 85, 297; for adolescents, 212; for children, 202–3; for cluster headaches, 176; as injections, 79, 174; for migraines, 74, 79, 85–86, 121, 132, 133, 202; nasal spray, 85, 196, 263; for older people, 222, 224, 225, 226. *See also* Ergotamine derivatives

DHE, intravenous (IV), 121, 124, 161, 162, 180, 185, 215, 223, 224, 231, 263

Diabetes, 226, 245, 262

Diamox, 102, 297

Diazepam, 84, 149, 151, 162. *See also* Valium

Diclofenac, 242

Diclofenac sodium, 157. *See also* Non-steroidal anti-inflammatories

Dihydroergotamine. See DHE

Dilantin, 297

Dilaudid, 297

Diltiazem, 116. *See also* Cardizem

Dimetapp, 288

Disalcid, 297

Ditropan, 297

Diuretics, 132, 134

Doan's Extra Strength, 286–87

Doctor: choice of, 43–45; relationship with, 42, 43–45, 48–51; and use of medication, xiv, 50, 122, 263

Dolobid, 297

Dolophine, 83, 161, 163. *See also* Methadone

Donnatal, 297–98

Dopamine, 261

Doral, 298

Doxepin, 108–9, 111, 155. *See also* Sinequan

Dramamine, 290

Dristan, 288, 298

Droperidol, 298

Drug therapy. *See* Medications for headache

Duradyne, 30

Duragesic-25/50/75/100, 298

Dura-Vent, 298
Duridren, 77. *See also* Midrin
Dyazide, 132, 134

Ear problems, 244
Eclectic Farms, 248
Ecotrin Enteric Coated Aspirin, 285, 298
Effexor, 15, 110–11, 111, 139, 156, 298
Effexor XR, 298
Elavil, 104, 106–7, 111, 154, 206, 213, 230, 298. *See also* Amitriptyline
Eldepryl, 298
Electroencephalogram (EEG), 48
Eletriptan, 71. *See also* Relpax
Emetrol, 87–88, 137, 290
Emotions, as migraine trigger, 95
Empirin aspirin, 284
Endorphins, 8, 22, 256, 257
Enkephalins, 256
Enteric aspirin, 284, 285
Entex LA, 298
Environmental factors, 5, 245, 264
Ephedrine. *See* Rynatuss
Epidural blood patch, 233–34
Epileptic seizure, 245
Equagesic, 299
Ercaf, 294
Ergocaf, 294
Ergomar, 78, 80, 132, 182, 222. *See also* Ergotamine tartrate
Ergonovine, 132, 133, 179, 182, 183, 299
Ergotamine(s): after age fifty, 139, 222, 225, 226; for cluster headaches, 176, 177, 179, 182–83; for migraines, 65, 78, 79–80; and rebound headaches, 8, 242; with triptans, 69, 70. *See also* Ergomar
Ergotamine derivatives, 132, 133
Ergotamine tartrate, 85, 132, 133, 174, 176
Ergotrate, 132, 133, 179, 183, 299. *See also* Ergonovine
Ergots, 138
Erythromycin, 299
Esgic, 65, 76, 77, 138, 149, 150, 165, 177, 201, 222, 299. *See also* Butalbital compounds
Esgic Plus, 65, 76, 149, 150, 299
Eskalith, 299
Essence Aromatherapy, 273
Estinyl, 135, 139, 299

Estrace, 135, 139, 299
Estraderm, 135, 299
Estradiol. *See at* Alesse; Ortho-Novum
Estratab, 299
Estratest, 299
Estratest HS, 299
Estrogen, 15, 101, 129, 130, 132, 135, 139, 242. *See also* Hormones
Ethinyl. *See at* Alesse; Ortho-Novum
Eucalyptus, 253
Evista, 299
Excedrin, Aspirin-Free, 31–32, 73, 196–97, 210, 282, 300
Excedrin Extra-Strength, 30, 32, 282, 286, 300; for adolescents, 210, 211; caffeine in, 28; for cluster headaches, 176; for migraines, 65, 73; for tension headaches, 146, 147
Excedrin Migraine, 30, 65, 73, 146, 147, 177, 210, 211, 222, 300
Excedrin PM, 282, 300
Excedrin Sinus, 288, 289
Exercise, 22, 101, 131, 239–40, 263
Exercise headaches, 14–15, 35, 231–33
Eye pressure test, 48
Eye problems, 244
Eyestrain headaches, 35, 193, 236–37

Family therapy, 194, 208
Fastin, 300
Fatigue, and migraines, 100
Fatty acids, long-chain, 252–53
Feeling Good: The New Mood Therapy (Burns), 36
Feldene, 300
Fenoprofen, 300
Fentanyl. *See* Duragesic
Feverfew, 117, 119–20, 158, 160, 214, 246, 247–48
Fevers, 243
Fibromyalgia, 254–55
Fibromyalgia Network, 274
Fioricet, 65, 76, 77, 138, 149, 150, 200, 201, 211, 222, 300. *See also* Butalbital compounds
Fioricet with codeine, 75, 77, 222, 300
Fiorinal, 65, 69, 70, 75, 77, 149, 150, 177, 200–201, 211, 222, 300; *See also* Butalbital compounds
Fiorinal with codeine, 75, 222, 300

Flexeril, 158, 159–60, 230, 300
Floralis, 274
Fluoxetine, 107, 111, 154–55. *See also* Prozac
Flurbiprofen, 115, 132–33, 157, 232. *See also* Ansaid
Food and Drug Administration (FDA), 11, 66, 136, 153, 198
Foods, 173, 235, 237; keeping track of, 35, 235, 264; and magnesium, 251; and MAO inhibitors, 122; as migraine triggers, 58, 95, 97–99, 131, 193–94, 251
Frovatriptan, 71

Gabapentin, 117, 119, 158, 214, 241. *See also* Neurontin
Gamma knife radiation, 187
Gastritis, and migraine medications, 66
Gelsemium, 254
Generic medications, 66, 75, 76–77, 84, 91
Genetic basis of headaches, 4–5, 56, 57, 261
Ginger, 247, 248
Gingko biloba, 250
Glaucoma, 47, 48
Glucotrol, 300
Glucotrol XL, 300
Glyburide, 300
Goody's Headache Powers, 300; Extra Strength, 284
Grapefruit juice, 86
Guaifenesin, 300
Guarana, 250

Halcion, 300
Haltran, 31, 146, 147, 286
Hangover headaches, 237
Hardening of the arteries, 67
Headache(s), xiii, 1–2, 262–64; after age fifty, 71, 118, 221–27; causes of, 5–7, 47, 56; cost of, 2; couples and families affected by, 15–16; and doctors' role, 2, 3; new-onset vs. long-standing, 231–32; as physical illness, 4–5; triggers of, 2, 7, 10, 35, 57 (*see also* Triggers of headaches); types of (common), 12–14; types of (less common), 14–15, 228–45. *See also* Medications for headache; Treatment; *and specific types*
Headache associations, 45, 267–80

Headache Intake Assessment Form, 45, 52–54
Head Injury Hotline, 279
Head scan, 46–47
Head trauma, 14, 102, 228–31
Health Messages, 268
Heart disease, 56, 124, 176, 243
Heart medications, headaches from, 15
Heart rate, and antidepressants, 106
Heat, as therapy, 33, 259
Hemicrania, chronic paroxysmal (CPH), 240, 241
Hemicrania continua, 239–40
Herbal Green Pages, 273
Herbal supplements, 41, 117, 119–20
Herb Companion Wishbook and Resource Guide, The (McRae), 273
Herb Research Foundation, 272
Herbs, ix, 38, 246–50, 263, 272–73
Herbs of Choice (Tyler), 247
Herb Society of America, 273
Herpes zoster, 241
High blood pressure, 47, 56, 112, 121, 124, 226, 244
Himalayan Institute of Yoga, Science, and Philosophy, 278
HIV headache, 243
Holiday headaches, 238–39
Homeopathy, 254
Hormonal therapy, 132, 134–36, 138–39
Hormones, 15, 35, 56, 129–41, 242
Hot tubs, 27
H2 blockers, 39
Hunger, 7, 58, 95, 100, 193, 245
Hycodan Syrup, 301
Hydralazine, 35
Hydrochlorothiazide, 132, 134
Hydrocodone, 137, 149, 150, 222. *See also* Vicodin
Hydrocodone with acetaminophen, 82
Hydro Duril, 301
Hydromorphone. *See* Dilaudid
Hydroxyzin, 301. *See also* Vistaril
Hygroton, 301
Hyoscyamine. *See* Cystospaz; Levsinex
Hypericum perforatum. See St.-John's-Wort
Hypertension. *See* High blood pressure
Hypnosis, 255, 277–78
Hypoglycemia, 245

Hypothalamus, 129, 171–72
Hytrin, 301

Ibuprin, 146, 147
Ibuprofen, 19, 31, 282–90, 301; for adolescents, 209, 210, 211, 213; for after-surgery headaches, 239; for children, 195, 197–98, 205, 206; for exertional headaches, 232; headaches caused by, 8, 242; for migraines, 64, 70, 72, 132–33; for post-traumatic headaches, 230; for tension headaches, 146, 147, 157; *See also* Advil; Motrin; Nonsteroidal anti-inflammatories
Ice, as headache therapy, 259
"Ice cream" headaches, 237
Imagery, 23
Imdur, 301
Imitrex, 9, 301; for adolescents, 211; as breakthrough medication, 119; for children, 196, 203; for cluster headaches, 174, 175, 176, 177, 183; for exertional headaches, 232; and MAO inhibitors, 122; for migraines, 64, 65, 67, 67–69, 70, 121, 125, 131, 132, 136, 139; for older people, 225; for post-traumatic migraines, 231; for tension headaches, 150, 151. *See also* Sumatriptan
Imitrex Nasal Spray, 67, 68, 91, 183, 203
Immune system, 235, 261
Imuran, 301
Inderal, 105, 112–13, 158, 159, 186, 205, 206, 230, 301. *See also* Propranolol
Indomethacin (Indocin), 179, 184, 232, 240, 301–2
Infections, headaches caused by, 243
Insight Publishing, 276
Institute for Brain and Immune Disorders, 280
International Association for the Study of Pain, 274
International Association of Yoga Therapists, 278
International Chiropractors Association, 280
International Imagery Association, 270
Iris, 254
Isocet, 302
Isollyl Improved, 302. *See also* Fiorinal

Isoptin, 105, 116, 158, 160, 181, 214, 302. *See also* Verapamil
IV DHE. *See* DHE, intravenous

Jaw clenching, 236
Jet lag, 245

Kadian, 121, 123, 161, 163, 263, 302
Kava kava, 38, 41, 247, 249–50
Ketoprofen, 33, 64, 72, 115, 132–33, 146, 147–48, 157, 211, 213. *See also* Nonsteroidal anti-inflammatories; OrudisKT
Ketoprofen, generic, 211, 213, 287
Ketorolac, 80–81; injections, 78, 80, 175, 177. *See also* Toradol
Kidney disease, and headaches, 56
Klonopin, 78, 84, 149, 151, 161, 162, 302

Lactation, 245
Lactic acid, 7
Lamictal, 302
Lavender, 253
Learned Optimism: How to Change Your Mind and Your Life (Seligman), 36
Levsinex Time Caps, 302
Librium, 149, 151, 161, 162, 302
Lidocaine, 240, 254
Lidocaine nasal spray, 175, 177, 188
Lifestyle strategies, 10
Light, and migraines, 58
Lights, bright, 35, 101
Limbitrol, 302
Lipitor, 302
Lithium, 106, 178, 179, 180, 181, 302
Lithobid Slow Release Tabs, 302
Lithonate, 302
Lithotab, 302
Liver, irritation of, 119
Lodine, 157, 302
Loestrin, 303
Lomotil, 303
Lo/Ovral, 303
Lopressor, 105, 113, 303
Lorcet, 82, 303. *See also* Narcotics
Lortab, 303
Lovastatin. *See* Mevacor
Lozenges, 85, 199, 203, 204
Lupron injections, 136, 304
Luvox, 304

Macrodantin, 304
Magnesium, 62, 251
Magnesium oxide, 117, 119, 120, 136, 304
Magnetic resonance imaging (MRI), 47
Magnet therapy, 259–60
MAO (monoamine oxidase) inhibitors, 110, 121–22, 161, 162, 186, 223, 249, 263
Marcaine, 240, 254
Marezine, 290
Marijuana, and adolescents' headaches, 219
Massage, 27, 258, 263, 277
Maxalt, 304; for adolescents, 211; for children, 196, 203; for cluster headaches, 175, 183; for exertional headaches, 232; and MAO inhibitors, 122; for migraines, 64, 65, 67, 69–70, 119, 121, 125, 131, 132, 136, 139, 231; for tension headaches, 150, 151
Meclizine, 304
Meclofenamate sodium, 132
Medical conditions, headaches caused by, 243–45
Medications: headaches induced by, 15, 35, 241–42; sinus, 235. See also Antinausea medications
Medications for headache, xiii–xiv, 3, 10, 16, 291–316; abortive, 9 (see also Abortive medications); accidental discovery of, 260; for adolescents, 209–15; for children's headaches, 195–203, 205–7; and choice of doctor, 44; for cluster headaches, 174–86; decision on strategy for, 9–10; for exercise headaches, 232–33; function of, 6–7; future possibilities in, 260–61; for migraines, 30, 64–86, 102–25, 132–36, 222–26; nonheadache uses of, 11; for occipital neuralgia, 241; over-the-counter, 10, 29–33, 281–90 (see also Over-the-counter pain relievers); and patient's role, xiv, 48, 50, 51, 63; for posttraumatic headaches, 230–31; preventive, 9, 63, 71, 90, 93, 139, 204–7, 208–9, 212–15; side effects of, xiv (see also Side effects); for tension headaches, 145–51, 152–63; use of, 262; as varying with situation, 216. See also Treatment

Medipren, 31, 146, 147. See also Ibuprofen
Meditation, 21–22
Medrol, 304. See also Depo-Medrol
Mellaril, 304
Meningitis, 12, 47, 243
Menopause, and migraines, 101, 138–39
Menstrual migraines, 101, 130–36; case study on, 140–41; corticosteroids for, 81; and hypothalamus, 129; and magnesium, 251; naproxen for, 71; and NSAIDs, 105, 114–15; triptans for, 70
Menstruation, 34, 35, 97
Meperidine, 83, 122. See also Demerol
Meridia, 304
Mesperidine, 137. See also Demerol
Metaxalone, 159. See also Skelaxin
Methadone, 78, 83, 121, 123, 163, 263, 304. See also Narcotics; Opioids
Methamphetamine, 121. See also Amphetamines
Methocarbamol, 160, 230. See also Robaxin
Methylphenidate, 163, 186, 263. See also Ritalin
Methysergide, 116, 118–19, 179, 181–82, 223. See also Sansert
Metoclopramide, 71, 87, 89. See also Reglan
Metoprolol, 113, 137. See also Lopressor
Mevacor, 305
Micomp, 294
Micronor, 305
Midol, 28, 30, 282, 305. See also Ibuprofen
Midol 200, 31, 146, 147, 305
Midrin, 9, 65, 74, 77, 146, 148, 195, 199–200, 211, 222, 305
Migraine Ice, 33, 259
Migraines, 12, 13, 55–59; in adolescents, 209, 211–12, 213–15; after age fifty, 221, 222–24; and AIDS, 243; aromatherapy for, 253; and auras, 12, 45, 57, 58, 59–60, 61, 62, 192; and blood pressure, 244; and blood-vessel sensitivity, 235; case studies on, 90–93, 125–28, 215–20; causes of, 61–62; and cervicogenic headache, 241; in children, 192, 193, 202; classical vs. common, 61; costs of, 55; and ear, 244; and hangover headaches, 237; and occipital neuralgia, 255; OTC medications for, 30; phases of, 60–61; physical basis of, 4–5; post-

traumatic, 228, 231; prevention of, 102–25, 260–61; psychological conditions with, 6; Saturday-morning, 238; and serotonin, 6, 62, 67, 96, 130; and sinus headaches, 234; and spinal tap headaches, 233; strategy for, 62–63; sufferers' reaction to, 172; and surgery, 239; and tension headaches, 142, 143, 144, 225; and tight-hat headaches, 238; transformed, 56; treatment of (in progress), 64–86; trigger-point injections for, 254; triggers of, 57, 58, 63, 94–102, 192, 193–94, 251; as vascular, 172; visual disturbances occurring with, 60; and vitamin B$_2$, 252; in women, 129–41

Migranal (DHE) Nasal Spray, 65, 74, 119, 133, 176, 196, 202–3, 212, 226, 305

Mind-Body Medical Institute, 275

Mineral remedies, 251–53

Mircette, 135

Mirtazapine, 110, 111

Mobigesic Analgesic Tablets, 287

Moduretic, 132, 134, 305

Monoamine oxidase (MAO) inhibitors, 110, 121–22, 161, 162, 186, 223, 263

Morphine, 78, 83, 163. *See also* Kadian; MS Contin; Narcotics

Motion, and migraines, 58, 102

Motrin, 8, 19, 31, 72, 146, 147, 157, 195, 197, 211, 232, 287, 305. *See also* Ibuprofen

MS Contin, 123, 161, 163, 305

MSG (monosodium glutamate), 97, 98, 173

"Muscle contraction headaches," 144

Muscle relaxants, 158, 159–60

Mylanta, 88

Nadolol, 113, 137, 159, 186. *See also* Corgard

Naprelan, 71, 105, 114–15, 157, 306

Naprosyn, 31, 105, 114–15, 157, 195, 199, 210, 306

Naproxen, 31; for adolescents, 210, 211, 213; for children, 195, 199, 205, 206; for cluster headaches, 177; for exertional headaches, 232; headaches caused by, 242; and hemicrania continua, 240; for migraines, 64, 71, 114–15, 118, 132–33; for older people, 222, 223; for

post-traumatic headaches, 230; for tension headaches, 145, 147, 157. *See also* Nonsteroidal anti-inflammatories

Naratriptan, 70. *See also* Amerge

Narcolepsy Network, 278

Narcotics: for cluster headaches, 174, 177; and headaches after age fifty, 222–23; for migraines, 65, 78–79, 81–84; for tension headaches, 148, 149, 150, 161, 163

Nardil, 110, 111, 122, 161, 162, 186, 215, 306. *See also* Phenelzine

Nasal sprays: and allergy, 235; DHE, 85, 196, 263; Imitrex, 67, 68, 183, 203; and migraines in women, 56, 129–41; lidocaine, 175, 177, 188; Migranal, 65, 74, 176, 196, 202–3, 212, 226, 305; and sinus/migraine, 235; Stadol, 78, 83, 311; sumatriptan, 174, 175

National Anxiety Foundation, 271

National Association of Social Workers, 270

National Brain Tumor Foundation, 280

National College of Naturopathic Medicine, 275

National Depressive and Manic-Depressive Association, 271

National Foundation for Depressive Illness, 271–72

National Headache Foundation, 55, 267

National Institute of Neurological Disorders and Stroke, 280

National Mental Health Association, 272

National Self-Help Clearinghouse, 268

National Sleep Foundation, 278–79

Natrum muriaticum, 254

Natural herbs/supplements, 117–20

Natural therapies, xv

Naturopathic medicine organizations, 274–75

Naus-a-way, 88

Nausea, 20, 25, 30, 58, 63, 66, 87–90

Nausea-tol, 88

Neck problems, causing headache, 241

Nefazodone, 111, 112. *See also* Serzone

Negative attitudes, coping with, 36–37

Nerve blocks, 255

Neuralgia, occipital, 240–41, 255

Neurological disorders, organizations on, 280

Neurontin, 117, 119, 158, 214, 223, 224, 241, 306

Nifedipine, 116, 186. *See also* Procardia
Nimotop, 306
Nitrates, 15
Nitroglycerin, 15, 242
Nitrous oxide, 261
NoDoz, 28, 74
Nolvadex, 132, 134, 306
Nonheadache medicines, 11
Nonsteroidal anti-inflammatories
   (NSAIDs), 29; with another medication,
   118, 161; and breastfeeding, 138; for
   children, 205, 206; headaches from, 15;
   for migraines, 64, 65, 71–72, 105,
   114–15, 132–33, 139; and nausea, 30;
   for older people, 223, 224, 225, 227;
   stomach problems from, 39, 118, 153;
   for tension headaches, 153, 156–57. *See
   also* Ibuprofen; Naproxen
Norco, 82
Norflex, 158, 160, 306
Norgesic, 306
Norgesic Forte, 9, 146, 148, 210, 306
Norpramin, 104, 110, 111, 155, 306
Nortriptyline, 109, 111, 155, 206, 207,
   213, 225, 230. *See also* Aventyl;
   Pamelor
NSAIDs. *See* Nonsteroidal anti-
   inflammatories
Nubain, 306
Nuprin, 8, 31, 72, 146, 147, 195, 197,
   287, 306. *See also* Ibuprofen
Nursing women, and feverfew, 248. *See
   also* Breastfeeding
NutraSweet, 99
Nux vomica, 254

Obsessive-Compulsive Foundation, 272
Occipital nerve blocks, 184, 241, 255
Occipital neuralgia, 240–41, 255
Odors, as headache trigger, 35
Office of Alternative Medicine, 274
Older people, headaches in, 221–27; and
   NSAIDs, 71, 118
Ondansetron, 87, 90. *See also* Zofran
Oophorectomy, 136
Opioids, 82, 84, 121, 123, 163, 186, 263.
   See also Narcotics
Oral Balance Gel, 107
Oral contraceptives, 242
Organic solvents, and migraines, 100

Organizations on headaches, 45, 267–80
Orphenadrine, 160. *See also* Norflex
Orphenadrine citrate, 210
Ortho-Novum, 306
Orudis, 115, 157, 307
OrudisKT, 33, 72, 105, 115, 146, 147–48,
   211, 213, 287, 307. *See also* Ketoprofen
Oruvail, 105, 115, 157, 213, 307
Osteopathy, organizations on, 277
Over-the-counter (OTC) pain relievers, 10,
   29–33, 281–90; for adolescents, 211; for
   children, 195; informing doctor of, 50,
   122, 263; and migraines, 63, 122; re-
   bound headaches from, 8, 56, 242; and
   tension headaches, 13
Oxycodone, 83. *See also* Oxycontin; Per-
   cocet; Percodan; Roxicet
Oxycontin, 78, 83, 121, 123, 161, 163,
   263, 307
Oxygen, for cluster headaches, 174,
   175–76, 177

P-A-C Analgesic Tablets, 286
Pacemaker, and magnets, 260
Pacific Institute of Aromatherapy, 273
Pain, 22, 46–47, 274
Paint, and migraines, 100
Pamelor, 109, 111, 155, 206, 213, 225,
   230, 307. *See also* Nortriptyline
Pamprin, 282, 307
Panadol, 282
Panic disorder, 106
Parafon Forte DSC, 307
Parlodel, 307
Paroxetine, 108, 111, 154–55. *See also*
   Paxil
Parthenolide, 247
Paxil, 15, 307; for children or adolescents,
   206, 207, 213, 214; and breastfeeding,
   138; for cluster headaches, 186; for mi-
   graines, 104, 106, 107, 108, 139; for
   older people, 224; for post-traumatic
   headache, 231; side effects of, 111; for
   tension headaches, 154–55
Peer groups, for adolescents, 194
People over fifty, 221–27, 71, 118
Pepcid, 39, 307
Pepcid AC, 307
Peppermint, 250, 253
Percocet, 78, 83, 307

Percodan, 78, 83, 307
Percogesic, 282, 307
Perfumes, 35, 100
Periactin, 186, 205, 307
Phenelzine, 110, 111, 122, 161, 162, 186, 215, 223, 224. *See also* Nardil
Phenergan, 69, 86, 87, 88, 91, 178, 204, 308
Phenergan with codeine, 307
Phenobarbital, 161, 162
Phentermine, 121, 124, 263, 308. *See also* Adipex-P; Fastin
Phone help, 268–70
Phrenilin, 65, 76, 77, 149, 150, 200, 201, 222, 223, 308. *See also* Butalbital compounds
Phrenilin Forte, 76
Physical therapy, 38, 258, 259
Physicians' Desk Reference, xiv, 50, 104, 242; for herbs, 247
Piper methysticum. See Kava kava
Placebo effect, 246
Platelets, 129
Post-traumatic headaches, 14, 102, 228–31
Posture, 259
Pravachol, 308
Prednisone, 78, 81, 131, 180, 196, 202, 261, 308. *See also* Cortisone
Pregnancy: and feverfew, 248; headaches during, 137; and kava, 249; and magnets, 260; and migraines, 101
Premarin, 139, 308
Premphase, 308
Prempro, 308
Presalin, 30
Prevacid, 39, 308
Preventive medication, 9, 262–63; for adolescents or children, 204–7, 208–9, 212–15; for cluster headaches, 178–85; for migraines, 63, 71, 90, 93, 102–25; for post-traumatic headaches, 230–31; for tension headaches, 152–63; and weight gain, 139
Prilosec, 39, 309
Procardia, 116, 186, 309
Prochlorperazine, 87, 88, 138, 178, 203. *See also* Compazine
Prodrome, 60
Progesterone, 15, 139, 242, 309. *See also* Premphase; Prempro; Provera

Progestin(s), 130, 139
Progressive relaxation training (PRT), 25
Promapar, 89. *See also* Chlorpromazine
Promethazine, 87, 88, 178, 204. *See also* Phenergan
Propoxyphene, 82, 149, 150. *See also* Narcotics
Propranolol, 112–13, 118, 137, 159, 161, 186, 205, 206, 223, 224. *See also* Inderal
Prostaglandins, 129
Proton pump inhibitors, 39
Protriptyline, 109, 111, 155, 213. *See also* Vivactil
Provera, 139, 309
Prozac, 15, 309; for adolescents' headaches, 213, 214; during breastfeeding, 138; for children's headaches, 206, 207; for cluster headaches, 186; for migraines, 106, 107, 109, 139; for older people's headaches, 224; for posttraumatic headaches, 231; during pregnancy, 137; side effects of, 111; for tension headaches, 154–55. *See also* Antidepressants
Pseudoephedrine, 281, 282–90
Psychotherapy, 35–37, 194, 263, 270–72

Quality of life, 16–17, 65
Quantum Quests, 269

Radiofrequency trigeminal rhizotomy, 187
Raloxifene. *See* Evista
Ranitidine, 39, 242. *See also* Zantac
Raynaud's syndrome, 116
Rebound headaches, 7–9, 145, 165, 242; from acetaminophen, 145; and caffeine, 8, 29, 98, 146, 147, 242; and migraines, 63; and transformed migraines, 56
Reflux (heartburn), 15, 38, 39
Reglan, 69, 71, 73, 86, 87, 89, 124, 137, 309
Relafen, 157
Relaxation, 19–27, 131, 145, 194, 208, 230, 263, 269–70
Relpax: for adolescents' headaches, 211; for children's headaches, 196, 203; for cluster headaches, 175; and MAO inhibitors, 122; for migraines, 64, 65, 67, 71, 121, 125, 132, 136, 139, 231; for tension headaches, 150, 151
Remeron, 15, 110, 111, 156, 309

Reserpine, 35
Respiratory illnesses, 56
Reye's syndrome, 200, 201
Riboflavin (vitamin B$_2$), 117, 119, 120, 136, 252
Risperdal, 309
Ritalin, 121, 124, 161, 163, 186, 309
Rizatriptan, 69–70. *See also* Maxalt
Robaxin, 158, 160, 230, 309
Robitussin A-C Syrup, 309
Rolaids, 31, 86, 88
Roxanol, 310
Roxicet, 309
Rufen, 31, 146, 147. *See also* Ibuprofen
Ru-Tuss, 310
Rynatuss, 310

S-A-C tablets, 30
St.-John's-Wort, 246, 249
St. Joseph Adult Chewable Aspirin, 284, 311
St. Joseph Aspirin-Free Fever Reducer for Children, 283
Salatin, 30
Saleto, 30
Sanguinaria, 254
Sansert, 116, 118–19, 179, 181–82, 223, 310
Seasonal change, 35, 100
Sedatives, 78, 84–85, 149, 151, 222
Self-help strategies, 18, 38; acceptance, 41; caffeine, 27–29; calendar, 34–35; cold and heat, 33; cool dark room, 34; over-the-counter pain relievers, 29–33; physical and chiropractic therapy, 38; psychotherapy and stress management, 35–37; relaxation and deep-breathing exercises, 19–27; and serious symptoms, 18–19; and sleep problems, 40–41; and stomach problems, 38–39
Self-hypnosis, 25–26, 255
Seligman, Martin E., 36
Sepia, 254
Serax, 310
Seroquel, 310
Serotonin, xiii, 4, 5–7, 261, 262; and antidepressants, 154, 205; and beta-blockers, 158; and blood vessels, 11; and caffeine, 27; and cluster headaches, 171; and magnesium, 251; and mi-graines, 6, 62, 67, 96, 130; and parthenolide, 247; and SSRIs, 138; and tension headaches, 13, 144; and TENS unit, 258; and tricyclic antidepressants, 106
Sertraline, 108, 111, 154–55. *See also* Zoloft
Serzone, 15, 110, 111, 112, 156, 310
Sex, 101, 107, 155, 259
Sexual headaches, 14–15, 232
Shingles, 241
Side effects: of abortive medications, 9; extrapyramidal, 88; headaches as, 241–42; of herbs, 247; need to inquire about, xiv; of OTC pain relievers, 30–31, 31, 32, 33; sexual, 107, 155
Sinarest, 288
Sine-Aid, 288, 310
Sine-Off, 288, 310
Sinequan, 104, 108–9, 111, 155, 310
Singulair, 261, 310
Sinus disease, 47
Sinus Excedrin, 288, 289
Sinus headaches, 14, 234–35
Sinus Medication, Tylenol, 289
Sinus x-ray, 47
Sinutab, 289, 310
Skelaxin, 158, 159, 311
Sleep, 38, 40–41; as headache trigger, 35, 95, 100, 101; regular schedule of, 264; and teenagers, 208
Sleep disorders organizations, 278–79
Smoke, 35, 100, 235
Smoking, 135–36, 172
Soma, 311
Sominex Pain Relief Formula, 282
Sonata, 311
Sonazine, 89. *See also* Chlorpromazine
Source Cassette Learning System, The, 269
Spinal tap, as diagnosis, 47–48
Spinal tap headaches, 233–34
Spine disorder, and headaches, 56
SSRIs (selective serotonin reuptake inhibitors), 138, 206, 207, 213, 224, 225, 231, 242
Stadol Nasal Spray, 78, 83, 311
Stemetic, 89
Steroid blockade, 180, 184
Steroids, 102, 138, 227
Stimulants, 121, 124, 263
Stomach problems, 38–39

Stress, 4, 5, 6, 20, 35–37, 263; in children or adolescents, 208, 217; as headache trigger, 35, 57, 58, 95–96, 131, 192; and stomach, 39; and weekend headaches, 238
Stretches, 258, 263
Stroke, 47, 136, 147, 221, 243–44
Sudafed, 289, 311
Sulfa antibiotics, 72
Sumatriptan, 9, 62, 67–69, 85, 122, 174, 175, 183. *See also* Imitrex
Sunglasses, 38, 58
Supac, 30
Support groups, organizations for, 268
Suppositories, 85, 199, 203
Surgery, 186–87, 239
Surmontil, 110, 111, 155–56, 311
Symptoms, serious, 18–19
Synalgos-DC, 311
Synthroid, 311

Tagamet, 39, 311. *See also* Cimetidine
Talacen, 311
Talwin, 311–12
Tamoxifen, 132, 134. *See also* Nolvadex
Tanacetum parthenium. See Feverfew
Tapes for relaxation, 27, 269–70
Tavist D, 312
Tavist Sinus, 312
Tebamide, 89. *See also* Trimethobenzamide
Tegamide, 89. *See also* Trimethobenzamide
Tegretol, 241, 312. *See also* Carbamazepine
Temporal arteritis, 226–27
Tenormin, 105, 113, 312
TENS (Transcutaneous Electrical Nerve Stimulation), 257–58
Tension (muscle-contraction) headaches, 12–13, 142–43; in adolescents, 209, 212–13; after age fifty, 221, 225; and aromatherapy, 253; and blood-vessel sensitivity, 235; case studies on, 163–70; and cervicogenic headache, 241; in children, 192; as inherited, 144; and migraines, 56; post-traumatic, 228; prevention of, 152–63; and serotonin, 6; and tight-hat headaches, 238; treatment for, 145–51; types of, 143
Testoderm Transdermal System, 312
Thorazine, 87, 89, 178, 312
Tic douloureux, 227

Ticon, 89
Tigan, 86, 87, 89, 203–4, 312
Tigect-20, 89
Tiger balm, 253
Tight-hat headaches, 237–38
Timolol, 113–14, 137
Tirend, 28
Tizanidine, 159. *See also* Zanaflex
TMJ (temporomandibular joint) headaches, 14, 236, 244
Tofranil-PM, 312
Topamax, 312
Toradol, 78, 80–81, 91, 141, 175, 177, 313
Tramadol, 82, 150. *See also* Ultram
Tranquilizers, 161, 162
Transient ischemic attack, 60
Tranxene, 313
Trauma, head, 14, 102, 228–31
Travel headaches, 35, 238
Treatment, 9–10; of adolescents' or children's headaches, 195–215; after age fifty, 222–26; alternative, 246–64; of cluster headaches, 173–87; diagnostic tests, 47–48; and doctor-patient relationship, 3, 10, 42, 43–45, 48–51; future possibilities, 260–61; infrequent use of, 3; of migraines, 62–63, 64–86, 130–36, 222–24; pain description, 46–47; and quality of life, 16–17; of tension headaches, 145–51, 152–63; trial-and-error, 3, 10–11, 63, 153; workups, 45–46. *See also* Medications for headache
Trendar, 31, 146, 147. *See also* Ibuprofen
Triamcinolone, 180. *See also* Cortisone
Triban, 89. *See also* Trimethobenzamide
Tribenzagan, 89. *See also* Trimethobenzamide
Tricyclic antidepressants, 106, 159, 161, 214
Trigeminal nerve, 62, 187, 234
Trigeminal neuralgia, 227
Trigesic, 30
Trigger-point injections, 254–55
Triggers of headaches, 2, 7, 10, 35; cluster headaches, 173–74; environmental factors as, 245, 264; as identifying headaches, 228; migraines, 57, 58, 63, 94–102, 131, 192, 193–94, 251; stress as, 35, 57, 58, 95–96, 131, 192
Trileptal, 313

Trimethobenzamide, 87, 89, 203–4
Trimipramine, 110, 111, 155–56. *See also* Surmontil
Tri-pain, 30
Triptans, 64, 65, 66–71; for children or adolescents, 196, 203, 211; after age fifty, 222; daily, 121, 124, 175, 179, 183, 263; for exercise headaches, 232; and MAO inhibitors, 122; for migraines, 131, 132, 136, 138, 139; for post-traumatic headaches, 231; for tension headaches, 150, 151
Tums, 31, 39, 86, 88, 124
TV, and children's headaches, 193
Tylenol, 8, 70, 72, 137, 145, 195, 283, 289, 313–14. *See also* Acetaminophen
Tylenol with codeine, 82, 163, 314
Tylenol PM, 283, 314
Tyler, Varro E., 247
Tylox, 78, 83, 314. *See also* Oxycodone

Ulcers, 15, 66
Ultram, 78, 82, 149, 150, 314
Unisom, 283

Valerian, 41, 247, 248
Valium, 78, 84, 149, 151, 161, 162, 222, 314
Valprin, 287
Valproate, 154, 161, 179, 213, 214, 224, 261. *See also* Depakote
Vanquish, 28, 30, 65, 73, 74, 283, 286, 314
Vascular headaches, 172
Vasoactive peptides, 261
Vasoconstrictor, 8, 235
Vasotec, 314
Venlafaxine, 110–11, 111
Verapamil, 116, 118, 160, 178, 179, 180, 181, 186, 214, 223, 224, 231, 242. *See also* Calan; Covera HS; Isoptin
Verelan, 105, 116, 158, 160, 181, 214. *See also* Verapamil
Vertigo, and migraines, 58
Vicodin, 69, 70, 78, 82, 137, 150, 163, 315. *See also* Hydrocodone
Vicoprofen, 78, 82, 315
Vioxx, 64, 71, 72, 105, 114, 115, 132, 146, 148, 156, 221–22, 222, 224, 227. *See also* Nonsteroidal anti-inflammatories
Vistaril, 315

Visualization, 23–24
Vitamin B_2, 117, 119, 120, 136, 252
Vitamin B_6, 87–88, 137, 252
Vitamin B_{12}, 252, 261
Vitamin C, 102
Vivactil, 104, 109, 111, 139, 155, 213, 315
Vivarin, 28
Voltaren, 105, 157, 315
Vomiting, 20, 58, 63, 217

Warm baths, 27
Water pills, 134
Weather changes, 35, 100
Web site, headache information on, ix, 267
Weekend headaches, 8, 29, 96, 238
Wellbutrin, 107, 110, 111, 139, 156, 315
Wigraine, 315
Willow bark, 250

Xanax, 315

Yoga, 27, 263; organizations on, 278

Zanaflex, 158, 159, 170
Zantac, 15, 39, 242, 315
Ziac, 315
Zithromax, 316
Zocor, 316
Zofran, 87, 90, 316
Zofran ODT, 90, 316
Zolmitriptan, 70. *See also* Zomig
Zoloft, 316; and breastfeeding, 138; as cause of headaches, 15; for children or adolescents, 206, 207, 213, 214; for cluster headaches, 186; for migraines, 104, 106, 108, 139; for older persons' headaches, 224; for post-traumatic headache, 231; and pregnancy, 137; side effects of, 107, 111; for tension headaches, 154–55, 213
Zolpiden. *See* Ambien
Zomig, 316; for adolescents' headaches, 211; for children's headaches, 196, 203; for cluster headaches, 175; for exertional headaches, 232; and MAO inhibitors, 122; for migraines, 64, 65, 67, 70, 119, 121, 125, 131, 132, 136, 139, 231; for tension headaches, 150, 151
Zydone, 82
Zyprexa, 316